Recent Advances in

Cardiolo

C000225431

Recent Advances in

Cardiology 17

Derek Rowlands BSc(Hons) MB ChB(Hons) MD FRCP FACC FESC
Honorary Consultant Cardiologist
Manchester Royal Infirmary, Manchester
Consultant Cardiologist
The Beeches Consulting Centre, Cheadle, UK

Bernard Clarke BSc(Hons) MBChB MD(Dist) FRCP(Lond) FRCP(Edin)
FESC FACC FRAeS FRCOG(Hon)
Honorary Clinical Professor of Cardiology
Institute of Cardiovascular Sciences, Manchester Academic Health
Science Centre, University of Manchester
Consultant Cardiologist
Manchester Royal Infirmary, Manchester, UK

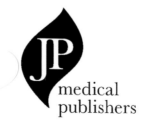

JP
medical
publishers

London • Philadelphia • Panama City • New Delhi

Preface

This latest volume of *Recent Advances in Cardiology* once more provides a range of important topics, written by highly experienced and internationally recognised authors. These authors have accepted the challenge of producing chapters which are brief but focussed, to accommodate the twin desires of this book, namely to be both supportive and challenging. Our aim is to form a bridge between rapidly published research reports and the subsequent consensus formed over time by experienced clinicians.

The topics included in this book all present everyday problems to the practising cardiologist or physician. All the chosen topics are in areas where there are still gaps in our knowledge, but we have been particularly fortunate in obtaining the services of authors who combine extensive experience in their field with fluency of communication.

Derek Rowlands
Bernard Clarke
July 2015

Contents

Chapter 1

The impact of South Asian ethnicity on the incidence and prognosis of coronary disease

M Justin Zaman

CORONARY MORTALITY BY ETHNICITY

Societies across the world experience different rates of various cardiovascular diseases, and within those societies, there exist differences among social class, gender and ethnicity. In the 1950s, studies from South Africa began to report differences in coronary disease rates between ethnic groups, in particular, between the South Asian group (predominately people originating from India, Bangladesh, Pakistan and Sri Lanka) and South Africans of other ethnicity. Shaper and Jones in 1959 stated that 'in the African population of Uganda coronary heart disease is almost non-existent. In the Asian community on the other hand coronary heart disease is a major problem' [1]. Adelstein in 1963 pointed out that among the South African ethnic types, people of Asian origin (almost entirely of Indian descent) showed the most unfavourable mortality rates from cardiovascular disease and that these rates were among the highest of the national rates on record in the world [2]. Subsequent UK studies of mortality also highlighted differences in the cause of death between different immigrant groups – 1991 census data revealed higher standardised mortality ratios for those born in South Asia (**Figure 1.1**) [3] and data from the 2001 UK census noted that though coronary mortality fell among migrants, rate ratios for coronary mortality remained higher for men and women from South Asia [4–6].

This chapter seeks to explain why there is a higher coronary mortality rate in South Asian than in white populations. The study of ethnic differences in health is of potential benefit not only to minority groups but also to the population at large around them, as the study of inequality in ethnic groups is a tool both for scientific analysis and for social action in the wider field of health inequalities [7]. Epidemiologically, the explanation for the higher coronary mortality in South Asian compared with white populations may either be a consequence of higher incidence of coronary disease in South Asian populations or a poorer prognosis of already-manifested coronary disease – or a combination of both. Evidence for the contributions of disease incidence and prognosis requires, respectively, incident events in 'healthy' cohort studies and examination of outcomes in clinical cohorts with manifest coronary disease.

M Justin Zaman MBBS MRCP PhD, Department of Cardiology, James Paget University Hospital, Gorleston-on-Sea, Norfolk, UK. Email: justinzaman@nhs.net (for correspondence)

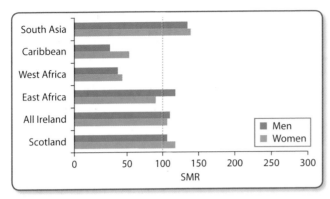

Figure 1.1 Standardised mortality ratios for coronary heart disease by sex and country of birth, 1989/92, England and Wales. Reproduced with permission from the British Heart Foundation [46].

A higher incidence in South Asian people (compared with white people) might be expected, as South Asian populations have a higher prevalence of insulin resistance and of diabetes mellitus than white populations [8], and this might lead to a higher incidence of subsequent coronary disease (**Table 1.1**). A worse prognosis might be expected owing to the fact that the presence of diabetes among those with coronary disease is itself associated with worse survival [9]. Furthermore, underuse of medical treatments (reported among South Asian patients by some [10,11] but not all [12,13] studies) might, in turn, adversely affect their survival, once they have presented with coronary disease (**Table 1.2**). South Asian patients with diabetes have poor knowledge and understanding of their disease which may also worsen their survival; in a cross-sectional survey of South Asian people living in South Tyneside comprised of 334 South Asian men and women aged 16–74 years, two-thirds of respondents said that, for both heart disease and diabetes, they did not understand enough about the conditions to prevent them [14]. The severity of disease at presentation may also be different between ethnic groups which would clearly influence their survival – South Asian patients have, e.g. been reported to have more severe angiographic coronary disease than whites when presenting with stable angina pectoris or acute coronary syndrome [15].

Table 1.1 Ethnic differences in coronary heart disease, risk factors and treatments between white and South Asian populations		
	South Asian	**White**
Coronary mortality rate	Higher	Lower
Incidence of diabetes	Higher	Lower
Age of the onset of diabetes	Younger	Older
Age of the onset of coronary disease	Younger	Older
Prevalence of smoking	High in Bangladeshis only	Equivalent to Pakistani South Asians, higher than Indian South Asians
Access to coronary intervention	Equivalent	Equivalent
Uptake of statin treatment	Higher	Lower
Prognosis of coronary disease	Better	Worse

Table 1.2 Key interventions recommended in reducing the inequality in coronary health between white and South Asian populations	
Issue	Solution for the health-care practitioner
Coronary mortality rates higher in South Asians Incidence of diabetes higher in South Asians	Focus on prevention – treat coronary risk factors earlier in South Asians.
Age of onset of diabetes younger in South Asians Age of onset of coronary disease younger in South Asians	Focus on prevention – treat coronary risk factors earlier in South Asians, with lifestyle interventions from childhood (especially in avoiding central obesity from diet and physical inactivity)
Prevalence of smoking higher in Bangladeshis	Target Bangladeshis in particular, but also be aware of the higher prevalence of smokeless tobacco products in all South Asian groups, in particular women
Access to coronary intervention equivalent	Maintain the status quo
Uptake of statin treatment higher in South Asians	Maintain the status quo if appropriate
Prognosis of coronary disease better in South Asians	Maintain the status quo

INCIDENCE OF CORONARY DISEASE IN SOUTH ASIANS COMPARED WITH WHITE POPULATIONS

Much of the work in this field at the turn of the century consisted of cross-sectional analyses of mortality statistics or cross-sectional surveys, as was found by a systematic review of this field published in the year 2000 [16] which retrieved 19 studies. There were very few cohort studies; none reported new disease incidence rates comparing the health of individuals in each ethnic group, and most of the review's retrieved studies reported prevalence, mortality rates or health-care utilisation data. Since this review, evidence from retrospective and follow-up of cross-sectional surveys (turning them into cohort studies) has been published. The paper by Fischbacher et al in 2007 [17] examined the incidence of fatal and nonfatal myocardial infarction through a record-linked, retrospective cohort study of 4.6 million people that linked individual ethnic group from the 2001 census to Scottish hospital discharge and mortality data from 2001 to 2003. The incidence of acute myocardial infarction (fatal combined with nonfatal) was higher in South Asian men compared with non-South Asian men, with a similar picture reported for women. Forouhi et al (2006) [18] also found a higher incidence of coronary death in 1420 South Asian men recruited in West London compared with 1787 European men. Furthermore, South Asian populations also have a higher incidence of earlier phenotypes of coronary disease. Over the 18-year follow-up of healthy civil servants in the Whitehall-II study, South Asian people had higher cumulative frequencies of typical angina (17.0% vs. 11.3%, $P < 0.001$) compared with whites [19]. It seems clear that there is a predisposition in South Asian people to develop metabolic abnormalities that lead to diabetes earlier and hence contribute to earlier and more incident coronary disease. However, where this emerges in the life cycle is not clear, nor it is yet clear what could be done about it.

PROGNOSIS OF CORONARY DISEASE IN SOUTH ASIAN PATIENTS COMPARED WITH WHITE PATIENTS

Is the prognosis of already-manifest coronary disease also worse in South Asian patients? The study of Fischbacher et al [17] also examined prognosis following myocardial infarction. After adjustment for age, sex and any previous admission for diabetes, the hazard ratio (HR) for death at 2 years was 0.59 (95% confidence interval (CI): 0.43, 0.81), reflecting a better survival among South Asian patients, a major surprise. Using a similar study design with routinely collected hospital administrative data linked to cardiac procedure registries from British Columbia and the Calgary Health Region Area in Alberta, Canada, Khan et al [20] reported that South Asian patients had a relatively lower risk of long-term mortality compared with white patients (HR: 0.65; 95% CI, 0.57–0.72). On the other hand, in-hospital and longer-term mortality of South Asian patients appeared no worse than that of whites as reported in a study of 9771 patients who underwent percutaneous coronary intervention in a London teaching hospital serving a large South Asian community (18.5% were South Asian, with diabetes being far more prevalent in these patients at 45.9% ± 1.2% vs. 15.7% ± 0.4%, $P < 0.0001$ in whites) [21].

COMPARING INCIDENCE WITH PROGNOSIS

This rather surprising survival advantage in South Asians was further underlined in a systematic review (the first in the South Asian cardiovascular disease field since Bhopal's in 2000 [16] and simultaneous meta-analysis which examined incidence alongside prognosis of coronary disease using old and more contemporary studies [22]. With regard to incidence of coronary disease in South Asian people compared with white people, from the studies included (11 incidence populations of 111,555 South Asians with 2527 events, 4,197,923 whites with 65,241 events) South Asians had a higher incidence of coronary disease compared with majority white populations (**Figure 1.2**, HR 1.35 (1.30–1.40)).

With regard to prognosis, meta-analysis of the studies that fitted the criteria of the review (12 prognosis populations;14,531 South Asian patients with 1591 events, 274,977 white patients with 63,758 events) showed that South Asian patients had a better prognosis from coronary disease compared with white patients (**Figure 1.3**, HR 0.78 (95% CI 0.74–0.82). These populations included a new cohort comprising all patients with acute coronary syndrome collected consecutively between 2004and 2008 from all 230 hospitals in England and Wales using the Myocardial Infarction National Audit Project (MINAP) [23]). The MINAP analyses allowed these researchers to investigate prognosis more carefully, and, in particular, the role of diabetes, receipt of secondary prevention medication at discharge, social deprivation and whether Indians, Pakistanis and Bangladeshis differed, respectively, compared with the majority white populations. Stratified analyses according to these demographic risk factors, disease phenotype and management characteristics showed that there were no strata in which South Asian patients had a worse prognosis than white patients. Thus, the better prognosis in South Asian patients could not be explained by differences in case mix, and the results appear to confirm those of others, as outlined above, that the prognosis of manifest coronary disease is no worse in South Asian patients than in white patients and may, in fact, be better.

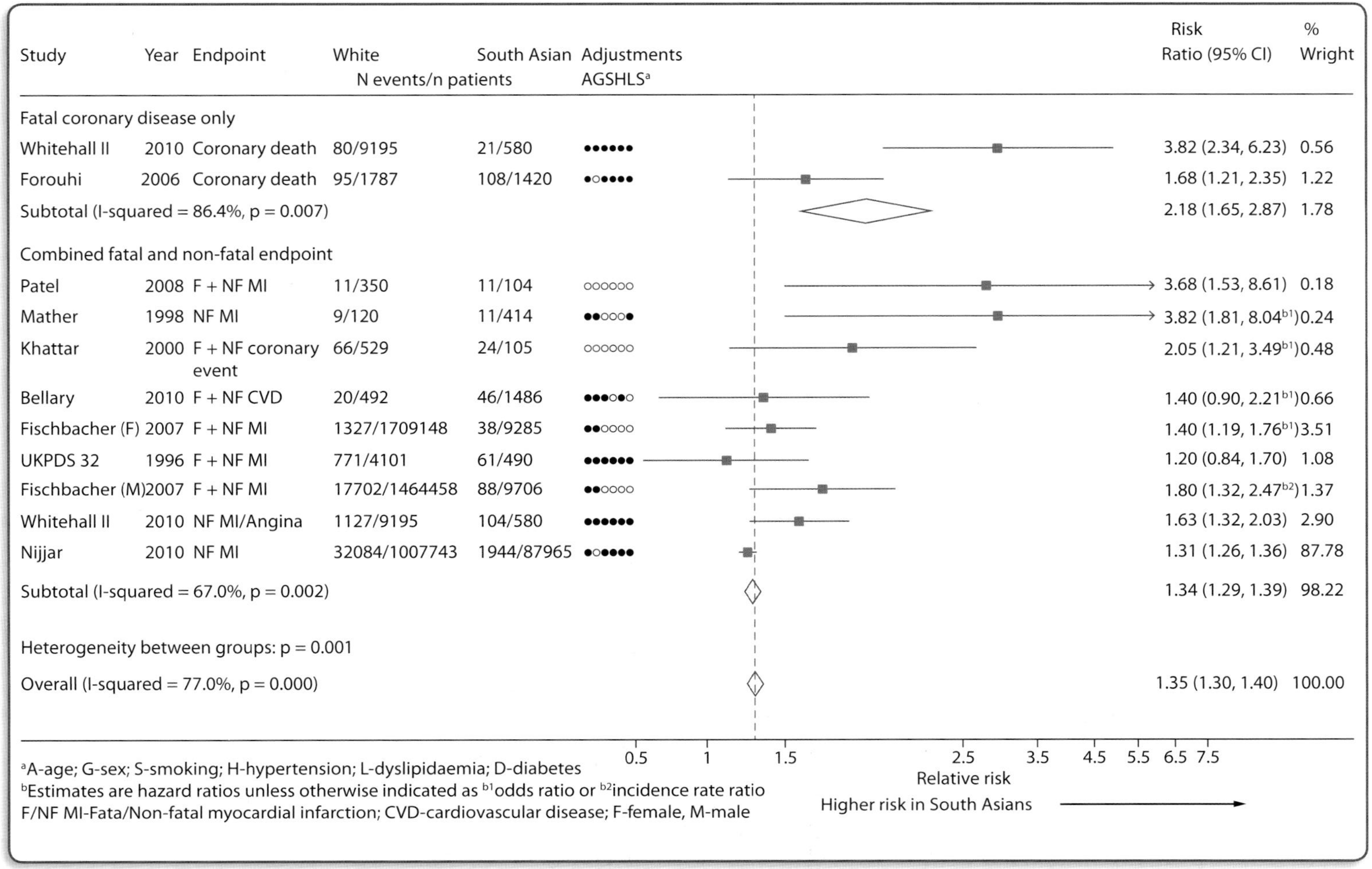
Study Year Endpoint White South Asian Adjustments Risk Ratio (95% CI) % Wright
N events/n patients AGSHLS[a]
Fatal coronary disease only
Whitehall II 2010 Coronary death 80/9195 21/580 ●●●●●● 3.82 (2.34, 6.23) 0.56
Forouhi 2006 Coronary death 95/1787 108/1420 ●○●●●● 1.68 (1.21, 2.35) 1.22
Subtotal (I-squared = 86.4%, p = 0.007) 2.18 (1.65, 2.87) 1.78
Combined fatal and non-fatal endpoint
Patel 2008 F + NF MI 11/350 11/104 ○○○○○○ 3.68 (1.53, 8.61) 0.18
Mather 1998 NF MI 9/120 11/414 ●●○○○● 3.82 (1.81, 8.04[b1])0.24
Khattar 2000 F + NF coronary event 66/529 24/105 ○○○○○○ 2.05 (1.21, 3.49[b1])0.48
Bellary 2010 F + NF CVD 20/492 46/1486 ●●●○●○ 1.40 (0.90, 2.21[b1])0.66
Fischbacher (F) 2007 F + NF MI 1327/1709148 38/9285 ●●○○○○ 1.40 (1.19, 1.76[b1])3.51
UKPDS 32 1996 F + NF MI 771/4101 61/490 ●●●●●● 1.20 (0.84, 1.70) 1.08
Fischbacher (M)2007 F + NF MI 17702/1464458 88/9706 ●●○○○○ 1.80 (1.32, 2.47[b2])1.37
Whitehall II 2010 NF MI/Angina 1127/9195 104/580 ●●●●●● 1.63 (1.32, 2.03) 2.90
Nijjar 2010 NF MI 32084/1007743 1944/87965 ●○●●●● 1.31 (1.26, 1.36) 87.78
Subtotal (I-squared = 67.0%, p = 0.002) 1.34 (1.29, 1.39) 98.22
Heterogeneity between groups: p = 0.001
Overall (I-squared = 77.0%, p = 0.000) 1.35 (1.30, 1.40) 100.00
0.5 1 1.5 2.5 3.5 4.5 5.5 6.5 7.5
Relative risk
Higher risk in South Asians
[a]A-age; G-sex; S-smoking; H-hypertension; L-dyslipidaemia; D-diabetes
[b]Estimates are hazard ratios unless otherwise indicated as [b1]odds ratio or [b2]incidence rate ratio
F/NF MI-Fata/Non-fatal myocardial infarction; CVD-cardiovascular disease; F-female, M-male

Figure 1.2 Incidence of coronary disease in South Asian compared with white populations. Reproduced with permission from BMJ Publishing Group Ltd. [47].

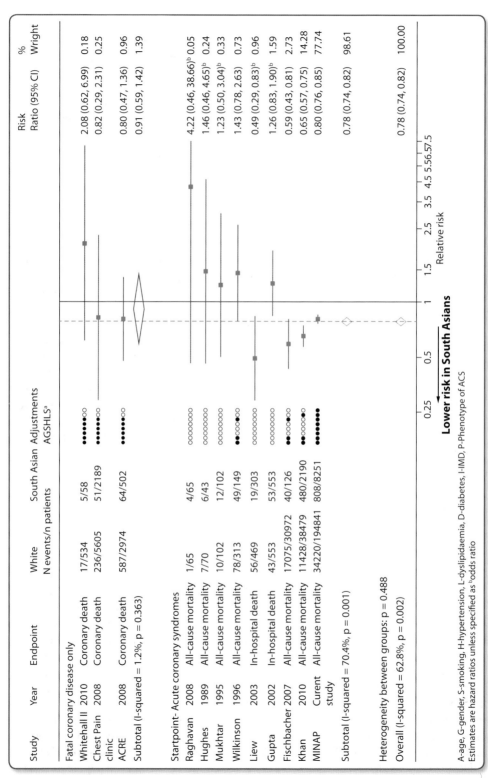

Figure 1.3 Prognosis of coronary disease in South Asian compared with white patients. Reproduced with permission from BMJ Publishing Group Ltd. [47].

The big news from the prognosis research area that is perhaps driving their more equitable future is that South Asian patients do not get worse health care – as once was the case and which is still widely thought to be so. The evidence suggesting better survival among South Asian patients suggests that – at least in studies of manifest coronary disease since the year 2000 – there is little contemporary evidence of ethnic inequities in health-care access and provision for cardiovascular health in the United Kingdom. Outcomes of out-of-hospital cardiac arrest in London are similar in South Asian people and other populations [24]. The introduction of pay for performance incentives in UK primary care has led to more equitable management of coronary disease across ethnic groups [25]. The 2001 Census and Quality and Outcomes Framework data suggest that statins, which play an important role in improving prognosis [26], are highly prescribed in South Asian patients – thus, this high-risk group is being addressed appropriately in the National Health Service [27].

The combination of higher incidence and equitable or even better prognosis in South Asian compared with white populations of coronary disease, coupled with the general aging of the whole UK population, will lead to an increase in the size of the prevalent pool of South Asian people. South Asian patients will also continue to suffer increased morbidity following presentation with acute coronary disease on account of their higher rates of diabetes and its ensuing complications and, since they present with coronary disease a decade earlier [22] than white people, this will lead to a less-compressed morbidity. Quality of life is likely to be worse in South Asian people partly due to their younger age of presentation with coronary disease (thus affecting work and family life) but also because they are less likely to get long-term relief from angina in comparison with white patients, as shown in a cohort of patients with angina undergoing coronary angiography where, again, prognosis in terms of subsequent events, such as myocardial infarction and death, was not worse in South Asian than in white patients [28]. As the relief of angina determines return to work and perceived health status, research on functional outcomes is of importance: as coronary mortality rates fall in all populations, morbidity in the form of angina becomes a more common clinical problem.

DRIVERS TO HIGHER INCIDENCE

Biological

The resulting conclusion is that in order for it to reduce persisting ethnic disparities in coronary mortality, a policy needs to be concentrated on reducing these inequalities in disease incidence (i.e. primary prevention). The increased prevalence of the metabolic syndrome and diabetes mellitus in South Asian populations is the most widely held explanation for the greater incidence of coronary disease and, though much of this excess is thought to be due to environmental factors, genetic factors may play a role in determining the level of such risk factors. An inherited susceptibility to type 2 diabetes may derive from multiple genes of individual modest effect [29], and a component of insulin resistance, more prevalent in South Asian populations [30], may be inherited [31]. The thrifty gene hypothesis proposes that conditions of food scarcity increased evolutionary selection pressure for efficient metabolism, which then troubles those who become exposed to the modern obesity-encouraging environment – the supposed combination facing the migrant from South Asia [32]. The influence of biological differences may continue adversely to affect not only South Asian migrants but also their children. South Asian populations have a smaller superficial subcutaneous adipose tissue compartment than white populations and a theory has been proposed that babies born to mothers of South Asian descent are smaller and have less peripheral fat, and that during subsequent growth and development, immersed in the richer diet of the developed world, this primary compartment reaches its capacity for fat storage rapidly and the deep subcutaneous and visceral compartments become more prominent, with adverse consequences for risks of diabetes and coronary disease [33]. Early evidence of ethnic differences in coronary risk has also been presented in a cross-sectional comparison of British South Asian and white children, such differences being present even in these children aged 8–11 years – an increased tendency to insulin resistance was observed in South Asian children, and the authors inferred an increased sensitivity to adiposity as a result [34].

Social

South Asians are comprised of different nationalities and religions (e.g. Indians, Pakistanis and Bangladeshis; Muslims, Sikhs and Hindus) and ideally all analyses comparing the health of this population with majority white populations should take this into account. However, the vast majority of studies that have presented results on ethnic differences between these two populations have used the aggregated 'South Asian' category, and those that collect data on the constituent peoples often do not have the power required for statistical analyses between South Asian peoples. The social heterogeneity of South Asian people becomes particularly important when comparing behavioural practices that may, in turn, determine a shift in future epidemiological disease patterns and may help to unravel reasons for the higher incidence of cardiovascular disease in these people. Bhopal et al cemented their arguments for disaggregating South Asian groups in the context of cardiovascular health by demonstrating huge differences in risk factor patterns in Bangladeshis (worst), Pakistanis (intermediate) and Indians (best) in Newcastle [35], and these findings have been backed up by analyses of data from the Health Surveys for England, showing that, for example, Bangladeshi men have much higher smoking rates (36%) than white men or, indeed, other South Asian groups [36] – Indian men smoked much less (15%) than all including white populations. Bangladeshis are shorter, less obese and have a lower mean blood pressure than other South Asian peoples, yet their risk of developing cardiovascular disease and diabetes is the highest of all the South Asian ethnic groups [37,38]. Much of the UK Bangladeshi community are classified as having low socioeconomic status, high rates of unemployment and low levels of formal female employment [39], and this social deprivation is one explanation for their higher smoking levels in these health surveys. Even allowing for the clear possibility of improvements in health care it seems likely that ethnic disparities in disease will remain as long as there are social disparities, especially those that are associated with cardiovascular risk factors.

Further evidence that ethnic differences in incidence of coronary disease may be more to do with social rather than biological factors can be inferred from a study of coronary mortality by specific country of birth across Denmark, England and Wales, France, The Netherlands, Scotland and Sweden. Previous work has focused mostly on the South Asian diasporas in the United Kingdom and Canada; hence this study presents data from countries from which South Asian ethnicity health and disease data have never been published. It showed that for most countries of birth groups – China, Pakistan, Poland, Turkey and Yugoslavia – there were substantial between-country differences [40], i.e. a Pakistani who migrates to Denmark has a rather different outcome from a Pakistani who migrates to Scotland. This emphasises that environmental, demographic and social factors influence disease occurrence in each national context beyond just skin colour. There are other high-income countries (such as Australia, Singapore, Norway and the United States) to which South Asian people migrate, and it is important to take this into account because some studies comparing the overall cardiac mortality of South Asian and white populations suggest a contextually specific relation according to the country of migration [40]. If, for example, immigrants are of higher education or skill status, their ability to integrate and adapt to the new country is better and they are likely to be less predisposed to the diseases of their new host country. Therefore, differences in the individual reasons for migration (e.g. economic, educational and political) and differences in baseline literacy and skills will result in heterogeneity of disease risk. Demobbed soldiers will be different from ship's cooks who will be different from doctors or others from professional and mercantile backgrounds. This will also influence the future socioeconomic and educational/professional status of their children, and thus disease risk. There is increasing evidence that those South Asian populations typically of the lowest socioeconomic status (Pakistani and Bangladeshi origin) have the highest rates of coronary disease [35,41]. It is thus a pertinent question to ask whether the sons and daughters of first-generation South Asian migrants will be at equal risk. In a study in Australia, decreasing mortality with increasing duration of residence in the new host country was observed for migrants from South Asia [42], perhaps due to cardioprotective behavioural practices practised by the more skilled nature of migrants there. In contrast, studies in the United Kingdom have opposing results, with cardiovascular risk among South Asian migrants to the UK increasing along with the duration of their residence [43]. The coronary risk of a group of educated and affluent second-generation South Asian people may more closely resemble that of a similarly educated and affluent white group, than that of a less-educated group and less-affluent group of second-generation South Asian people. It could, perhaps, be that the heterogeneity of the South Asian group will become increasingly important in the future. It is interesting that, apart from Indian people, minority ethnic groups (including Pakistani and Bangladeshis) are found to be more likely than majority white groups to engage in poor dietary behaviours in a study of adolescent and parental lifestyles, with those born in the United Kingdom and girls being particularly susceptible [44]. Therefore, some South Asian people may inherit the diseases of their parents more through their behaviour than through their genes.

The INTERHEART study suggests that the socioeconomic contribution to disease aetiology in South Asians is potentially stronger than any biological predisposition [45]. The South Asia component of this international case–control study recruited 1732 patients presenting with their first acute myocardial infarction alongside 2204 controls matched by age and sex from 15 medical centres in 5 South Asian countries, and showed that the majority of risk in these native South Asians could be explained by 9 potentially modifiable risk factors with similar collective impact as in other countries. The authors concluded that the earlier age of myocardial infarction in South Asian populations was a result of their higher risk factor levels at a younger age, as ethnic origin was the same for all who took part in this study. What was interesting here was that this paper was examining South Asian people who had not migrated to richer countries, and showing that conventional risk factors were associated with coronary disease in the same way as they were in the developed world. This paper thus suggested that concentrating on ethnicity alone was a wrong approach; considering that Bangladeshis in Bangladesh had the highest prevalence for most risk factors among the controls (e.g. smoking at 59.9%) and the lowest prevalence for regular physical activity (1.3%), the paper infers that coronary disease is caused by lifestyle and behaviour wherever you live, irrespective of your ethnicity. The marked variation in age of presentation of myocardial infarction in South Asians, with Bangladeshis being the youngest and Nepalese the oldest, indicated further that the onset of incident coronary disease can be delayed by modifying risk factors rather than having to worry about modifying biology.

CONCLUSION

Recent literature has revealed that although incidence of coronary disease is higher in South Asian compared with white populations, the prognosis of clinically manifest coronary disease in South Asian compared with white patients may be better now. This is probably driven by increasingly equitable, if not better, access to health care, but may also be due to the younger age of presentation of disease in South Asians which may remain a confounder that cannot be fully adjusted away. It is clear that South Asians have a greater predisposition to cardiometabolic dysfunction but that the risk factors that finally lead to incident coronary disease are well-established ones, applicable to all ethnic groups. Furthermore, adverse risk profiles within South Asian individuals may be driven by community-level socioeconomic drivers. Thus, the answer is earlier prevention (compared with white populations), and this means preventing the adoption of lifestyles that raise risk. Modification of risk factors and behaviour should take place from school onwards for South Asians and continue through to adulthood, and via high-risk population approaches (e.g. in deprived communities). If not addressed, then the combination of higher incidence and similar prognosis in South Asian compared with white populations of coronary disease, coupled with the general aging of the whole UK population, will lead to an increase in the size of the prevalent pool of South Asian people with coronary disease. Therefore, although coronary mortality rates may continue to drop, the total burden of coronary heart disease in South Asian populations is likely to increase.

Key points for clinical practice

- Coronary mortality in the United Kingdom is highest for men and women than from South Asia.
- South Asian populations have a higher prevalence of diabetes mellitus than white populations.
- South Asians have a higher incidence of coronary disease compared with white populations.
- South Asians increasingly have a better prognosis from coronary disease compared with white populations.
- There is little contemporary evidence of ethnic inequities in health-care access and provision for cardiovascular health in the United Kingdom.
- South Asian populations continue to suffer increased morbidity following disease presentation.
- South Asians comprise different nationalities and religions with marked heterogeneity between them.
- Ethnic differences in coronary health may be more to do with social rather than biological factors.

REFERENCES

1. Shaper AG, Jones KW. Serum-cholesterol, diet, and coronary heart-disease in Africans and Asians in Uganda. Lancet 1959; 2:534–537.
2. Adelstein AM. Some aspects of cardiovascular mortality in South Africa. Br J Prev Soc Med 1963; 17:29–40.
3. Wild S, McKeigue P. Cross sectional analysis of mortality by country of birth in England and Wales, 1970–92. BMJ 1997; 314:705.
4. Harding S, Rosato M, Teyhan A. Trends for coronary heart disease and stroke mortality among migrants in England and Wales, 1979–2003: slow declines notable for some groups. Heart 2008; 94:463–470.
5. Wild SH, Fischbacher C, Brock A, Griffiths C, Bhopal R. Mortality from all causes and circulatory disease by country of birth in England and Wales 2001–2003. J Public Health (Oxf) 2007; 29:191–198.
6. Fischbacher CM, Steiner M, Bhopal R, et al. Variations in all cause and cardiovascular mortality by country of birth in Scotland, 1997–2003. Scott Med J 2007; 52:5–10.
7. Bhopal R. Ethnicity, race, and health in multicultural societies; foundations for better epidemiology, public health, and health care. Oxford: Oxford University Press, 2007.
8. Barnett AH, Dixon AN, Bellary S, et al. Type 2 diabetes and cardiovascular risk in the UK south Asian community. Diabetologia 2006; 49:2234–2246.
9. Malmberg K, Yusuf S, Gerstein HC, et al. Impact of diabetes on long-term prognosis in patients with unstable angina and non-Q-wave myocardial infarction: results of the OASIS (Organization to Assess Strategies for Ischemic Syndromes) registry. Circulation 2000; 102:1014–1019.
10. Sekhri N, Timmis A, Chen R, et al. Inequity of access to investigation and effect on clinical outcomes: prognostic study of coronary angiography for suspected stable angina pectoris. BMJ 2008; 336:1058–1061.
11. Feder G, Crook AM, Magee P, et al. Ethnic differences in invasive management of coronary disease: prospective cohort study of patients undergoing angiography. BMJ 2002; 324:511–516.
12. Britton A, Shipley M, Marmot M, Hemingway H. Does access to cardiac investigation and treatment contribute to social and ethnic differences in coronary heart disease? Whitehall II prospective cohort study. BMJ 2004; 329:318.
13. Jones M, Ramsay J, Feder G, Crook AM, Hemingway H. Influence of practices' ethnicity and deprivation on access to angiography: an ecological study. Br J Gen Pract 2004; 54:423–428.
14. Rankin J, Bhopal R. Understanding of heart disease and diabetes in a South Asian community: cross-sectional study testing the 'snowball' sample method. Public Health 2001; 115:253–560.
15. Silbiger JJ, Stein R, Roy M, et al. Coronary artery disease in South Asian immigrants living in New York City: angiographic findings and risk factor burdens. Ethn Dis 2013; 23:292–295.
16. Bhopal R. What is the risk of coronary heart disease in South Asians? A review of UK research. J Public Health (Oxf) 2000; 22:375–385.
17. Fischbacher CM, Bhopal R, Povey C, et al. Record linked retrospective cohort study of 4.6 million people exploring ethnic variations in disease: myocardial infarction in South Asians. BMC Public Health 2007; 7:142.
18. Forouhi NG, Sattar N, Tillin T, McKeigue PM, Chaturvedi N. Do known risk factors explain the higher coronary heart disease mortality in South Asian compared with European men? Prospective follow-up of the Southall and Brent studies, UK. Diabetologia 2006; 49:2580–2588.
19. Zaman MJ, Shipley MJ, Stafford M, et al. Incidence and prognosis of angina pectoris in South Asians and Whites: 18 years of follow-up over seven phases in the Whitehall-II prospective cohort study. J Public Health (Oxf) 2011; 33:430–438.
20. Khan NA, Grubisic M, Hemmelgarn B, et al. Outcomes after acute myocardial infarction in South Asian, Chinese, and white patients. Circulation 2010; 122:1570–1577.
21. Jones DA, Rathod KS, Sekhri N, et al. Case fatality rates for South Asian and Caucasian patients show no difference 2.5 years after percutaneous coronary intervention. Heart 2012; 98:414–419.
22. Zaman MJ, Philipson P, Chen R, et al. South Asians and coronary disease: is there discordance between effects on incidence and prognosis? Heart 2013; 99:729–736.
23. Herrett E, Smeeth L, Walker L, Weston C. The Myocardial Ischaemia National Audit Project (MINAP). Heart 2010; 96:1264–1267.
24. Shah AS, Bhopal R, Gadd S, Donohoe R. Out-of-hospital cardiac arrest in South Asian and white populations in London: database evaluation of characteristics and outcome. Heart 2010; 96:27–29.
25. Millett C, Gray J, Wall M, Majeed A. Ethnic disparities in coronary heart disease management and pay for performance in the UK. J Gen Intern Med 2009; 24:8–13.

26. Ferrieres J, Cambou JP, Gueret P, et al. Effect of early initiation of statins on survival in patients with acute myocardial infarction (the USIC 2000 Registry). Am J Cardiol 2005; 95:486–489.

27. Ashworth M, Lloyd D, Smith RS, Wagner A, Rowlands G. Social deprivation and statin prescribing: a cross-sectional analysis using data from the new UK general practitioner 'Quality and Outcomes Framework'. J Public Health 2007; 29:40–47.

28. Zaman MJ, Crook AM, Junghans C, et al. Ethnic differences in long-term improvement of angina following revascularization or medical management: a comparison between south Asians and white Europeans. J Public Health (Oxf) 2009; 31:168–174.

29. McCarthy MI, Hattersley AT. Learning from molecular genetics: novel insights arising from the definition of genes for monogenic and type 2 diabetes. Diabetes 2008; 57:2889–2898.

30. Anand SS, Yusuf S, Vuksan V, et al. Differences in risk factors, atherosclerosis, and cardiovascular disease between ethnic groups in Canada: the Study of Health Assessment and Risk in Ethnic groups (SHARE). Lance2000; 356:279–284.

31. Kooner JS, Baliga RR, Wilding J, et al. Abdominal obesity, impaired nonesterified fatty acid suppression, and insulin-mediated glucose disposal are early metabolic abnormalities in families with premature myocardial infarction. Arterioscler Thromb Vasc Biol 1998; 18:1021–1026.

32. Neel JV, Weder AB, Julius S. Type II diabetes, essential hypertension, and obesity as 'syndromes of impaired genetic homeostasis': the 'thrifty genotype' hypothesis enters the 21st century. Perspect Biol Med 1998; 42:44–74.

33. Sniderman AD, Bhopal R, Prabhakaran D, Sarrafzadegan N, Tchernof A. Why might South Asians be so susceptible to central obesity and its atherogenic consequences? The adipose tissue overflow hypothesis. Int J Epidemiol 2007; 36:220–225.

34. Lampe FC, Morris RW, Walker M, Shaper AG, Whincup PH. Trends in rates of different forms of diagnosed coronary heart disease, 1978 to 2000: prospective, population based study of British men. BMJ 2005; 330:1046.

35. Bhopal R, Unwin N, White M, et al. Heterogeneity of coronary heart disease risk factors in Indian, Pakistani, Bangladeshi, and European origin populations: cross sectional study. BMJ 1999; 319:215–220.

36. Karlsen S, Millward D, Sandford A. Investigating ethnic differences in current cigarette smoking over time using the health surveys for England. Eur J Public Health 2012; 22:254–256.

37. Gill PS, Kai J, Bhopal RS, et al. Health care needs assessment: black and minority ethnic groups. In: Raftery J, Stevens A, Mant J (ed). Health Care Needs Assessment. The epidemiologically based needs assessment reviews. Third Series. Abingdon: Radcliffe Publishing Ltd, 2007.

38. Hippisley-Cox J, Coupland C, Vinogradova Y, et al. Predicting cardiovascular risk in England and Wales: prospective derivation and validation of QRISK2. BMJ 2008; 336:1475–1482.

39. Eade J, Vamplew T, Peach C. The Bangladeshis: the encapsulated community. In: Peach C (ed.), Ethnicity in the 1991 census. London: HMSO, 1996:150–160.

40. Bhopal RS, Rafnsson SB, Agyemang C, et al. Mortality from circulatory diseases by specific country of birth across six European countries: test of concept. Eur J Public Health 2011; 22:359-364.

41. Bhopal R, Hayes L, White M, et al. Ethnic and socio-economic inequalities in coronary heart disease, diabetes and risk factors in Europeans and South Asians. J Public Health 2002; 24:95–105.

42. Gray L, Harding S, Reid A. Evidence of divergence with duration of residence in circulatory disease mortality in migrants to Australia. Eur J Public Health 2007; 17:550–554.

43. Harding S. Mortality of migrants from the Indian subcontinent to England and Wales: effect of duration of residence. Epidemiology 2003; 14:287–292.

44. Harding S, Teyhan A, Maynard MJ, Cruickshank JK. Ethnic differences in overweight and obesity in early adolescence in the MRC DASH study: the role of adolescent and parental lifestyle. Int J Epidemiol 2008; 37:162–172.

45. Joshi P, Islam S, Pais P, et al. Risk factors for early myocardial infarction in South Asians compared with individuals in other countries. JAMA 2007; 297:286–294.

46. Allender S, Peto V, Scarborough P, et al. Coronary heart disease statistics, 2006 edition. London; British Heart Foundation, 2006.

47. Zaman MJS, Philipson P, Ruoling C, et el. South Asians and coronary disease: is there discordance between effects on incidence and prognosis? Heart 2013; 99:729-736.

Chapter 2

Sudden and/or unexpected cardiac death in young adults

Derek Rowlands

INTRODUCTION

Sudden cardiac death (SCD) is always a distressing event. Sudden unexpected cardiac death (SUCD) in the young inevitably brings a greater degree of poignancy and leads to questions about the possibility of having been able to prevent it, to predict it, or at least of having been able recognise its possibility in the person concerned. Clinically recognisable causes, such as hypertrophic cardiomyopathy (HCM), aortic stenosis and long QT syndrome (LQTS), are examples which, to differing degrees, can sometimes be recognised in the asymptomatic subject, but the overall situation is very complex, and most cases of SCD in the young are not currently predictable. The issue is so important, and uncertainties about how to minimise the incidence are so great that, in the USA in October 2013, the National Institutes of Health and the Centers for Disease Control and Prevention announced the setting up of a collaborative registry to estimate the incidence of sudden death in infants, children and young adults.

DEFINITIONS

The term 'young adult' is not usually precisely defined and there is no clear consensus on the definition of SCD (e.g. the terms 'sudden cardiac death' and 'sudden cardiac arrest' are often used interchangeably) [1]. This makes it difficult to derive consistent conclusions from the variety of studies available. For the purposes of this discussion, the following definitions have been chosen.

Sudden cardiac death

This may reasonably be defined as natural death from known or suspected cardiac causes occurring within 1 h of the onset of an abrupt change in cardiovascular status [2A].

Sudden unexpected cardiac death

This may be defined as SCD occurring in those subjects not known to have any predisposing cause. Thus, for example, patients known to have LQTS who die suddenly would fall into the

Derek Rowlands BSc MB ChB MD FRCP FACC FESC, Manchester Royal Infirmary, Manchester, UK. Email: djr@djr12ecg.demon.co.uk (for correspondence)

category of SCD but not into that of SUCD. On the other hand, those with LQTS undiagnosed at the time of sudden death would come under the heading of SUCD [2B].

Young adults

For the purposes of this chapter, this term has been defined as those within the age range from 14 to 35. However, a minor degree of flexibility in this definition has been assumed in order to encompass a variety of the very heterogeneous studies available.

INCIDENCE

It is particularly difficult to be sure of this most important and fundamental statistic. Reported data may be from observational studies, autopsy studies, local community analysis, retrospective death certificate analysis, etc. The lack of total consensus, between the various studies, concerning the definitions referred to above, adds to the difficulty. In the United Kingdom, the incidence of SCD in the young is thought to be in excess of 400 per year [3]. Bastiaenen and Behr have pointed out that the commonest scenario relates to young men dying in their sleep or at rest and that only in a minority of cases is there a history of prior syncope [4].

One of the most useful and disciplined studies is that from King County (Washington) [5] in which, at the time of the study, approximately 50% of the population (of 620,000) were ≤35 years old. This was a retrospective analysis of a cohort of 361 cases (305 of which were in the 14–35 age range) of out of hospital cardiac arrest (OHCA) over a period from 1980 to 2009. Data were obtained from autopsy reports, death certificates, emergency service reports and from all available medical records. This study concluded that the risk of OHCA was 1 in 69,000 persons per year in the age group 14–24 and 1 in 23,000 for the age group 25–35. Over the 30-year period of the study, the average annual incidence rates (per 100,000 persons) of OHCA were 1.44 for ages 14–24 and 4.4 for ages 25–35. Unsurprisingly, in the first 2 years of life, congenital cardiac abnormalities were found to constitute the largest group (84%) of cases of OHCA. Nonhereditable cardiomyopathies (dilated cardiomyopathy and myocarditis) made a relatively uniform contribution within the age range 3–35 (ages 3–13, 11%, ages 14–24, 18%, ages 25–35, 13%). HCM and LQTS appeared to have their greatest impact in the 3–13 age range. Perhaps the most striking finding was that, within the 25–35-year age group, coronary artery disease accounted for almost half (43%) of cases of OHCA.

POPULATION BURDEN AS OPPOSED TO DIAGNOSTIC GROUP INCIDENCE

The population burden of SCD in relation to any causative factor is given by the product of (i) the prevalence of SCD within the group of those holding that factor and (ii) the prevalence of that factor in the population as a whole. Thus, while the prevalence of SCD is far higher in a given group of persons with, say, arrhythmogenic right ventricular cardiomyopathy (ARVC) than in a similar-sized group of persons with no clinical or investigational (resting ECG, exercise ECG, etc.) evidence of any cardiac abnormality, the absolute number of persons in the latter category unknowingly predisposed to coronary disease is so large that the product of this and the (low) prevalence of SCD in that group gives rise to a much larger population burden of SCD from this cause. This paradox has very major implications when it comes to considerations about the best way forward in terms of reducing the population incidence of SCD. Thus, in population terms, it may well be more effective to address the question of known coronary risk factors in the apparently healthy young population than to seek out that tiny part of the population with potentially unstable cardiac rhythms.

CONDITIONS PREDISPOSING TO SUCD IN YOUNG ADULTS

The range of possible causes of SUCD in the young is considerable, but five main aetiological groups can be recognised. These are (1) congenital cardiac abnormalities, (2) inheritable cardiomyopathies, (3) 'electrical' syndromes associated with a clear disposition to cardiac arrhythmias, (4) premature coronary disease and (5) dilated cardiomyopathies and myocarditis. The impact of congenital heart disease is greatest in those <14 years old. Congenital anomalies of the coronary arteries (CCAs) represent the exception to this rule. CCAs (predominantly anomalous origin of the left main coronary artery from the right coronary sinus or the origin of the right coronary artery from the left coronary sinus) are rarely detected in children and can be the cause of sudden death in young adults (especially in athletes). Premature coronary disease is a significant cause of SUCD in young adults. The predisposing factors are, of course, well recognised. Dilated cardiomyopathies and myocarditis are usually (though not always) clinically apparent. These patients predominantly present with symptoms of ventricular dysfunction, so when sudden death occurs it is not usually totally unexpected. Furthermore, there is no clear age predominance. For these reasons, these conditions are discussed here only briefly.

The main groups of conditions to be considered are as follows.
1. Inheritable cardiomyopathies
   a. Hypertrophic cardiomyopathy (HCM)
   b. Arrhythmogenic right ventricular cardiomyopathy (ARVC)
2. 'Electrical' syndromes with a clear predisposition to arrhythmias
   a. Long QT syndromes (LQTS)
   b. Short QT syndromes (SQTS)
   c. Brugada syndrome (BrS)
   d. Catecholaminergic polymorphic ventricular tachycardia (CPVT)
   e. Wolff–Parkinson–White syndrome (WPW)
3. Coronary artery problems
   a. Congenital coronary anomalies (CCA) and premature coronary disease
4. Dilated cardiomyopathy

Any condition in the first three groups may have SCD as the first event or may be discovered by chance, by the screening of affected relatives, by clinical assessment following the complaint of palpitations, dizziness or syncope or after a successfully treated or spontaneously aborted SCD. Data predicting the possibility of preventing SCD through screening procedures are very limited [6]. SCD represents 75% of all fatalities during exertion [7] and this represents one category where screening can be helpful. Occult coronary disease, unsuspected prior to the SCD is, in numerical terms, the most common predisposing factor, i.e. it presents the greatest population burden.

SCD IN INHERITABLE CARDIOMYOPATHIES

Hypertrophic cardiomyopathy

HCM is characterised by inappropriate (i.e. without a predisposing cause) hypertrophy of the left ventricular myocardium with cellular disarray. The condition has a clear predisposition to the development of ventricular tachydysrhythmias.

Prevalence and genetics

This condition is the commonest genetically determined cardiomyopathy. The prevalence appears to be about 0.2% in the general population, a figure which seems to be similar in different parts of the world [8]. It is thought that this may well be an underestimate of the true prevalence since it is known that many of those with the condition remain asymptomatic and many do not have any major reduction in life expectancy.

Approximately 1500 mutations involving >11 genes have been demonstrated [9]. The condition has an autosomal dominant inheritance pattern. Each offspring, therefore, has a 50% chance of developing the disease, but the penetrance is age dependent with the majority presenting during adolescence or in teenage years.

SCD in HCM

HCM is one of the commonest causes of SCD in people under 30 years of age in the United States and is the commonest cause of SCD in athletes. However, the condition is compatible with a normal life expectation. Maron et al [10] studied 312 consecutively enrolled patients at the Minneapolis Heart Institute. Approximately 25% lived to an age of 75 or beyond and, of these, 60% lived to ages of 80–96. Importantly, for those patients aged 50 years or older at the time of diagnosis, the survival at 5, 10 and 15-year post-diagnosis did not differ significantly from that of a matched general population. Soraja et al [11], in a study of 544 consecutive asymptomatic or minimally symptomatic patients, in the age range 59 ± 16 years, showed only a minimal excess mortality (69.3% 10-year survival vs. 71.9% anticipated survival) and 46% of the observed deaths were due to noncardiac causes.

The ECG in HCM

The ECG is abnormal in about 90% patients with HCM and in about 75% of asymptomatic close relatives [12], but the abnormalities do not correlate with the severity of HCM as determined by echocardiography [8]. A wide variety of abnormal configurations occur, the commonest being the QRS and S–T,T changes of left ventricular hypertrophy, with increased QRS voltages, ST depression and T wave inversion. Counterintuitively, sometimes there may be reduced R wave voltages in the left precordial leads (**Figure 2.1**). One common feature of the ECG in HCM is the finding of prominent q waves. The usual criteria for an abnormality of abnormal q wave (in leads other than cavity leads) are a duration of ≥0.04 s or a magnitude of >25% of the ensuing R wave in two contiguous leads. The mechanism of the development of q waves in HCM is different from that in myocardial infarction and best criteria for abnormality of q waves in HCM involve q waves >3 mm in depth and/or >0.04 s in duration in at least two leads, excluding aVR [13,14]. An example is shown in **Figure 2.1**. About 6% patients with clear echocardiographic evidence of HCM have a normal 12-lead ECG at the time of diagnosis and these patients appear to have a less severe phenotype and a better outcome [15].

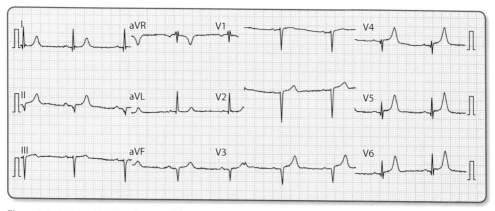

Figure 2.1 A 12-lead ECG in a 54-year-old asymptomatic patient with proven hypertrophic cardiomyopathy. The appearances do not indicate left ventricular hypertrophy (though this was unquestionably demonstrated by echocardiography). Abnormal Q waves are seen in leads V_1 to V_5 and in II, III and a VF. The patient did not have coronary disease.

Risk factor stratification in HCM

In 2011 a guideline for the diagnosis and treatment of hypertrophic cardiomyopathy was published by the American College of Cardiology Foundation/American Heart Association Task Force on Practice Guidelines, giving detailed recommendations concerning risk assessment and management of patients with HCM. The first is that patients remaining completely asymptomatic to beyond the age of 50 have an excellent prognosis [10]. The second is that implantable cardioverter defibrillator (ICD) placement is recommended for patients with HCM who have experienced a documented cardiac arrest, ventricular fibrillation (VF) or haemodynamically significant ventricular tachycardia (VT; level of evidence B) [8]. Patients proven to have HCM should not participate in intensive, competitive sporting activity [16].

Arrhythmogenic right ventricular cardiomyopathy

This is an inherited cardiomyopathy predominantly affecting right ventricular myocardium, with fibrofatty replacement of areas of myocardium creating a fertile substrate for the development of ventricular arrhythmias. The patients may present with syncope, palpitations, VT or supraventricular arrhythmias (including atrial fibrillation). Occasionally, right (or, even less commonly, left) ventricular failure can occur, but the commonest mode of presentation is SCD.

Prevalence and genetics

This is a hereditable condition afflicting young adults, most commonly presenting in the age range 10–40. The general prevalence is thought to be 0.02–0.1% [17]. Five desmosomal genes have been identified [18]. Most commonly the inheritance pattern is autosomal dominant with incomplete penetrance and variable phenotypical expression [18]. Familial occurrence is observed in 30–50% cases [17]. A particular variant of the condition, associated with palmoplantar keratosis and woolly hair, is found in Naxos and in other Hellenic islands.

SCD in ARVC

Of all the cardiomyopathies, ARVC is the one most likely to cause SCD (HCM being the second most likely). ARVC is usually both asymptomatic and occult before the teenage years and SCD is the most common initial presentation. High-level exercise substantially increases the risk of SCD in these patients, and there is clear evidence that endurance exercise and frequent exercise both increase the risks of VT, VF and SCD in desmosomal mutation carriers [18]. Although it is a cardiomyopathy, and in its terminal stages there may be all the manifestations of congestive cardiac failure (including atrial fibrillation and thromboembolism), in the main its manifestations are those of VT and SCD.

The ECG in ARVC

The 12-lead ECG is often highly informative in patients with this condition, although it may be entirely normal at presentation. The main findings during sinus rhythm are (1) precordial T wave inversion, (2) epsilon waves, (3) prolongation of the QRS duration in right precordial leads not matched in V_6 and (4) a right bundle branch block (RBBB) pattern. Of these, the commonest finding is of T wave inversion. T wave inversion in V_1 and V_2 is normal in infancy and T wave inversion in V_1 can persist throughout life, but the T wave is normally upright in V_2 by age 12. The T waves in V_2 were always upright in adult males and usually upright in adult females in the series studied by Macfarlane and Lawrie [19]. In apparently healthy adults, the T wave is always upright in V_3 [19]. **Figure 2.2** (a) shows an example of a 12-lead ECG from a 48-year-old woman with ARVC. **Figure 2.2** (b) shows a 12-lead ECG of a patient with ARVC during an episode of VT. The ECG findings are diagnostic of a tachycardia arising from the right ventricular outflow tract.

Risk factor stratification in ARVC

Large, prospective studies to demonstrate the unequivocal significance of presumed risk factors in this condition are not currently available. However, features thought likely to be associated with increased risk of SCD include prior cardiac arrest, syncope (particularly when exertion-related), demonstrated episodes of VT, young age at presentation and intense physical exercise. There is evidence that both endurance exercise and frequent exercise increase age-related penetrance Patients proven to have ARVC are advised not to participate in intensive, competitive sporting activity [16].

SCD IN THE 'ELECTRICAL' SYNDROMES

The so-called 'electrical' syndromes are those in which there is a marked predisposition to the development of cardiac arrhythmias in the absence of any accompanying morphological pathology. The WPW syndrome necessarily has a morphological abnormality [the congenital presence of an accessory pathway (AP)], but it has no pathological morphology and is conveniently considered within this group.

Inherited long QT syndromes

These are inherited conditions characterised by prolongation of the QT interval on the ECG and associated with the occurrence of syncope or of sudden death, usually on the basis of ventricular arrhythmias, most particularly via *torsades de pointes*.

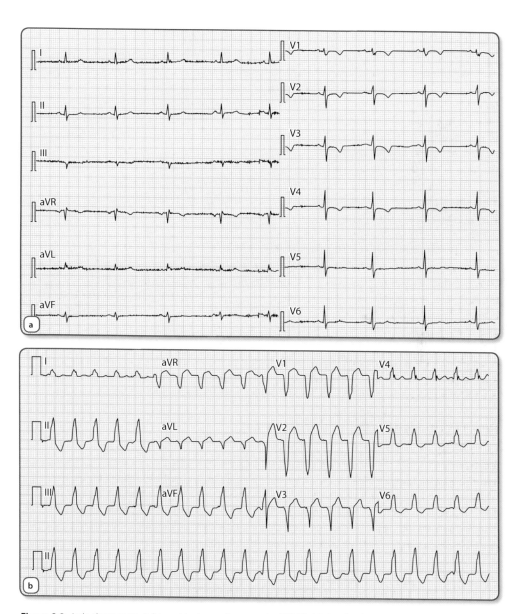

Figure 2.2 Arrhythmogenic right ventricular cardiomyopathy (ARVC). (a) A 12-lead ECG in a female patient aged 48, with arrhythmogenic right ventricular cardiomyopathy. There is T wave inversion from V_1 to V_4 and the T waves are abnormal in V_5. Epsilon waves are seen in the terminal part of the QRS complexes in V_1. (b) An example of right ventricular outflow tract tachycardia in a (different) patient with ARVC. The finding of atrioventricular dissociation with a ventricular rate greater than the atrial rate (well seen in the lead II strip) is diagnostic of ventricular tachycardia (VT). The QRS complexes have a perfect left bundle branch block configuration, indicating that the tachycardia originates high up on the right side of the interventricular septum. The frontal plane QRS axis in the VT is $+75^0$ indicating the arrhythmias arises at the base of the heart. Beyond dispute, therefore, this is a right ventricular outflow tract tachycardia.

Prevalence and of inherited long QT syndromes

Inherited LQT syndromes are uncommon conditions resulting from inherited cardiac channelopathies associated with prolongation of the QT interval of the ECG and a clear predisposition to ventricular arrhythmias, dizziness, syncope and sudden death. The overall prevalence appears be somewhere in the region of 1:2000 of the population [20]. It is thought to be one of the commonest causes of autopsy negative unexpected sudden death in young adults [21].

The vast majority of LQTS are inherited in an autosomal-dominant pattern. The exception is the Jervell and Lange–Nielsen syndrome in which the inheritance pattern is autosomal recessive. To date >500 mutations of 13 different genes have been recognised as the basis of LQTS [22]. More than 95% of these mutations are responsible for the first three types (LQT1, LQT2, LQT3).

Syncope and sudden cardiac death in LQTS

The range of possible presentations and of outcomes in those with the LQT phenotype is considerable. Those with the condition may remain asymptomatic or may present with fainting, syncope or sudden death. Schwartz has emphasised that many may run a very benign course [23].

The ECG in LQTS

By definition, all types of LQTS have prolongation of the QT interval, but there are major differences in the morphology of the ST segments and the T waves. In LQT1, the T waves begin early after the QRS and are broad based; in LQT2, the T waves are of low amplitude and often notched or bifurcated; and in LQT3 the T waves begin late after the QRS (i.e. there is a long ST segment) and are narrow (**Figure 2.3**).

Rate correction of measured QT intervals

The QT interval varies inversely as the heart rate and comparisons of observed QT readings with perceived normal values are made after 'rate correction' of the observed values (to give 'QTc'), most commonly, following the application of the Bazett formula. However, it is well recognised that this formula overcorrects at all values for the heart rate other than 60 bpm, the overcorrection being positive (i.e. giving inappropriately long QTc values) when the heart rate at the time of observation is above 60 and negative (i.e. giving inappropriately short QTc values) when the heart rate at the time of observation is <60. The greater the rate deviation from 60 bpm, the greater the adjustment (positive or negative) produced by the any correction formula and the limitations of 'rate correction' should be borne in mind when the observed heart rate is outside the range 50–80 [24].

Technique of measurement

QT interval measurement is far from straightforward and even arrhythmia specialists are prone to error in this area. QT interval measurement should, therefore, be made in a consistent and logical fashion. Measurements should be made manually: they should be made from a high-quality 12-lead ECG with the recording frequency set at 0.05–150 Hz; the lead showing the longest QT measurement should be used; it should be acknowledged that the reliability of predictions made on rate-corrected values is questionable when the heart rate is (1) irregular, (2) changing or (3) outside the range of 50–80 per minute [24].

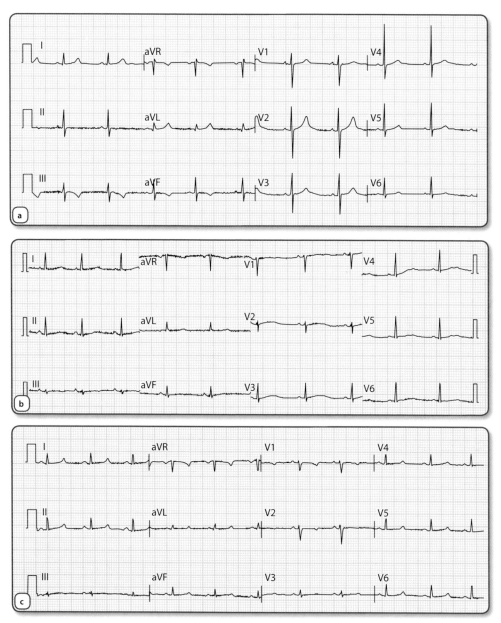

Figure 2.3 The three commonest phenotypes of the long QT syndrome (LQTS). (a) LQT1: the T waves begin early after the QRS complexes and are broad. (b) LQT2: the T waves are of low voltage and are not readily distinguishable from the U waves. (c) LQT3: the T waves begin late and are narrow.

Normal limits for QTc

It should be emphasised that LQTS is primarily a clinical rather than an electrocardiographic diagnosis. The important factors to be taken into account are (1) the mode of presentation, (2) the previous personal history, (3) any relevant family history (e.g. of proven LQTS or of syncope, or SCD) and (4) the ECG. A significant proportion (probably, about one-third) of patients with genetically proven LQTS have borderline or normal QTc measurements so LQTS cannot be excluded on the basis of a normal value for QTc. No simple classification of 'normal' and 'abnormal' QTc values has been universally agreed upon. Complex scoring systems have been suggested, but for general clinical use a simple stratification is required. Issa et al [22] suggest values as given in **Table 2.1**. It should be noted that there is considerable variability in serial QT interval measurements made in those with LQTS (there are sometimes diurnal variations) and the longest observed measurement should be used in patient assessment. Issa et al stress that, unless the value exceeds 500 ms, the QTc interval should always be assessed together with the other diagnostic criteria (including scoring systems) [22].

Risk stratification in LQTS

The strongest predictors of SCD in patients with LQTS are (1) previous aborted cardiac arrest and (2) repeated or recent unexplained syncope. The risk is also related to age, gender phenotype and environment. Over the age of 14, females generally have a higher risk than males, with LQT2 females carrying the highest risk, LQT1 females having an intermediate risk, and males with LQT1 and LQT2 having the lowest risk [25]. In patients with LQT1, the greatest likelihood of cardiac events is during stress or exercise. In patients with LQT2, the events most commonly occur during sudden auditory stimulation or sudden stressful events, particularly, when occurring against a background of rest, relaxation or sleep (e.g. when being woken by the alarm, by the telephone ringing or by any sudden noise). In keeping with these well-recognised features beta-blockers are recommended for all high-risk patients with LQT1 and LQT2 (unless contraindicated) as first-line therapy. In patients with LQT3, cardiac events are most likely to occur during sleep or relaxation (without auditory or other stimuli). The 36th Bethesda Conference recommendations [16] are that patients with LQTS of any phenotype or genotype should avoid all competitive sports (except category 1A sports) if they have previously experienced a suspected LQTS precipitated syncope or cardiac arrest, and that, in particular, phenotype negative, but genotype positive persons should not take part in competitive swimming.

The special case of Jervell and Lange–Nielsen syndrome

This is the most severe of the LQT syndromes with the majority of sufferers experiencing cardiac events, often at a very young age. It is much less common than the other forms of LQTS (because of its autosomal recessive inheritance pattern), is associated with

Table 2.1 Normal, abnormal and borderline abnormal QTc values in men and women [22]		
Probable normality or otherwise of the observed QTc value	**QTc (Men)**	**QTc (Women)**
QTc definitely prolonged* (i.e. these values are hardly ever seen in healthy individuals)	>470	>480
LQTS can be suspected	>450	>460
LQTS very unlikely	<390	<400
*Provided acquired forms of LQT have been excluded, these values are considered diagnostic of LQTS.		

congenital deafness and typically presents problems in infancy and early childhood. It will, therefore, not be discussed further here.

Short QT syndromes

The SQTS was first described in the year 2000 and very few families with this condition have so far been studied. Patients may present with syncope, SCD or atrial fibrillation and the QTc is usually <360 ms. The general principles of management are as for those with LQTS.

Brugada syndrome (BrS)

This is associated with characteristic, but time-varying ST segment elevation in right precordial leads, unexplained by structural organic heart disease, myocardial ischaemia or electrolyte disturbance and with a high incidence of ventricular arrhythmias and sudden death [26]. The condition is inherited via autosomal dominance, but sporadic cases can occur. Cases may present with syncope, cardiac arrest or death, may be revealed accidentally (e.g. by a preoperative ECG) or may be discovered following the recognition of the condition in a close relative. Arrhythmic events revealing this condition have been recorded as occurring from the ages of 2 days to 84 years [27].

Prevalence and genetics of BrS

The prevalence of this condition is certainly low, but it is difficult to be sure of the precise prevalence since its existence is only revealed by (1) the unexpected occurrence of ventricular arrhythmias, syncope or (aborted) sudden death, (2) an ECG from a family member presenting in that way or (3) an ECG fortuitously recorded for some other reason. The ECG is clearly the key to the diagnosis, but it is essential to be aware of the fact that the ECG appearances can change dramatically within minutes (**Figure 2.5**). It is clear that the prevalence is not the same in different geographical areas. The highest prevalence (both in relation to the ECG findings and sudden unexpected death) is in Asia where the type 1 ECG appearances are seen in 0–0.36% of the population [26]. The corresponding figures relating to Europe and to the United States are, respectively, 0–0.25% and 0.03% [25].

The mode of inheritance is that of an autosomal dominant pattern (with incomplete penetrance). About >250 mutations involving 7 genes have so far been identified [4].

Those with the typical ECG appearances of BrS (type 1 ECG Brugada pattern – *vide infra*) often remain completely asymptomatic. Patients may present with a mistaken diagnosis of epilepsy or may have laboured nocturnal respiration. SCD from BrS can occur at any age, the peak incidence being in the age range 30–50. SCD in those with BrS typically occurs at rest or during sleep, particularly during the early hours of the morning when there is a background of sinus bradycardia. It appears to be significantly more likely after a heavy meal or during a pyrexia and may be precipitated by alcohol or by various drugs, including cocaine (http://www.brugadadrugs.org).

Diagnosis of BrS

The diagnosis of BrS is based on the combination of two criteria:
1. Type 1 Brugada ECG pattern (with or without infusion of a sodium channel blocking agent) in one or more of the six parasternal leads (*vide infra*)
   Type 2 or type 3 Brugada ECG pattern, changing to type 1 with provocative drug testing in one or more of the six parasternal leads (*vide infra*) [20]
   and

2. One or more of the following [22]:-
    a. documented VF
    b. documented polymorphic VT
    c. family history of SCD at age below 45 years
    d. coved-type ECG in family members
    e. inducibility of VT with programmed electrical stimulation
    f. syncope without a clear explanation
    g. nocturnal agonal respiration

ECG in BrS

Three 'Brugada patterns' are recognised (**Figure 2.4**), but only one of these (type 1) is the specific Brugada pattern which, in combination with one or more of the items listed in the preceding paragraph, suffices to give the diagnosis of BrS.

The characteristic (type 1) Brugada pattern (**Figure 2.4**) is seen in the parasternal leads and consists of ≥2 mm of coved [i.e. convex (seen from above)] ST segment elevation, which continues, without any isoelectric interval, into a negative T wave. There may be a broad secondary R wave in these leads immediately prior to the onset of the elevated ST segment but, when present, this is not accompanied by a broad late S wave in the left precordial leads, as in typical RBBB. The QRS duration is, therefore, often slightly longer in V_1 than in V_6. In the standard 12-lead ECG, the appearances may be seen in the two parasternal leads, V_1 and V_2.

The use of additional recording of leads V_1 and V_2 in the third and second intercostal spaces, giving a total of 6 'parasternal leads' (*vide supra*) increases the sensitivity in respect of recognising the presence of a type 1 pattern [27]. Currently, the criterion for the diagnosis of 'Brugada ECG' is the recognition of the type 1 pattern, with ST elevation of 2 mm or more in one or more of the six parasternal leads, either occurring spontaneously or following provocation by intravenous Class 1 antiarrhythmic drugs [20]. The diagnosis is also justified when type 2 or type 3 Brugada pattern is found in one or more of the six parasternal leads only if the pattern converts to type 1 on intravenous administration of Class 1 antiarrhythmic drugs [20].

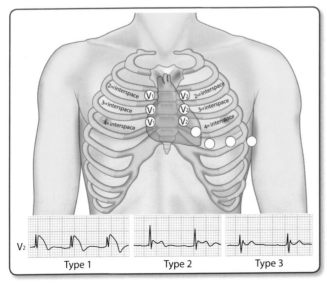

Figure 2.4 Recording positions from which diagnostic appearances may be observed and the three Brugada patterns. The upper part shows the positions of the six parasternal leads. These are conventional leads V_1 and V_2 plus similar leads placed one and two intercostal interspaces higher. The lower part shows the three types of Brugada pattern as described in the text. Only the finding of type 1 pattern contributes to the definitive diagnosis of Brugada syndrome.

It is important to be aware of the great variability of the ECG appearances in patients with BrS. Dramatic variation can occur on a beat-to-beat basis as shown by the ambulatory ECG recording in **Figure 2.5**.

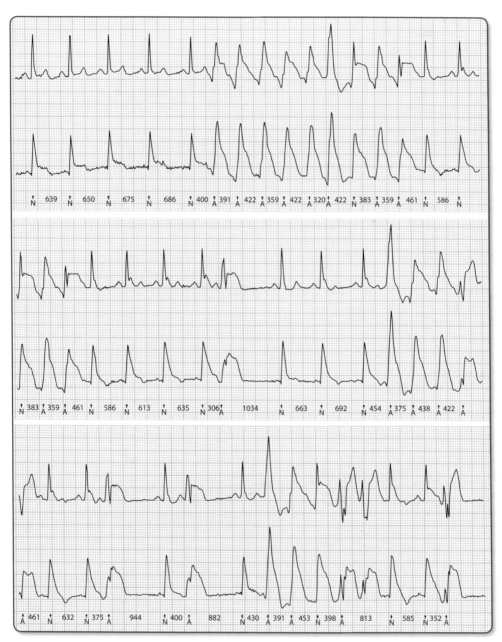

Figure 2.5 Striking variation in the form of the QRS complexes and of the ST segments occurring within a period of 13 s. The patient remained asymptomatic during this recording. ECG courtesy of Professor Bernard Clarke, Manchester Academic Health Science Centre, Manchester, UK.

Risk stratification in BrS

The most significant risk predictor in a patient with BrS is the record of a prior cardiac arrest. All such patients require an ICD. The second most significant risk predictor is a history of syncope or of demonstrated VT. Risks are higher in those patients presenting initially with a clear spontaneous type 1 ECG pattern and perhaps especially so in those demonstrating fragmentation of the QRS complexes [28], though this is an uncommon finding. Male patients carry a higher risk than females.

Catecholaminergic polymorphic ventricular tachycardia

This is an inherited arrhythmogenic condition with a very high incidence of sudden death in those affected. It is thought that >60–80% of patients experience syncope or cardiac arrest before the age of 40 [29]. The commonest presentation is in children or teenagers. Exercise and emotional stress are both powerful factors in the initiation of arrhythmias in this condition.

Prevalence and genetics of CPVT

There is no precise information on the prevalence of this condition, but it is rare. The majority of familial cases show an autosomal dominant inheritance pattern with a very small minority showing an autosomal recessive pattern.

ECG in CPVT

The resting 12-lead ECG is usually completely normal in this condition. Prominent U waves are sometimes seen in the right-sided chest leads, the T waves may be notched or bimodal and U wave variability ('U wave alternans') may be seen during the recovery period after an exercise ECG but CPVT cannot be diagnosed from the resting 12 lead ECG, which is typically entirely normal in this condition. More importantly, ambulatory ECG recordings may reveal frequent ventricular and/or atrial premature beats, runs of ventricular or of atrial tachycardia, atrial fibrillation or the typical bidirectional tachycardia – a dramatic alternation between two different frontal plane QRS axes (**Figure 2.6**). All of these rhythms are more likely to occur during exercise testing and the finding of atrial and ventricular ectopic activity progressively increasing with greater levels of exercise and leading to bidirectional VT is very highly likely to indicate CPVT.

Risk stratification in CPVT

Precise risk stratification is not possible because of the small number of cases reported, but the overall mortality rate is high. Early age of onset, prior syncope, exertion-related syncope and the occurrence of increasingly frequent and complex arrhythmias with increasing levels of physical activity are all bad prognostic signs. Treatment with beta-blockers is recommended in all symptomatic patients and ICD implantation is recommended in all those with CPVT who experience syncope or show bidirectional VT while on maximally tolerated doses of beta-blockers [20].

Wolff–Parkinson–White syndrome

The diagnosis of WPW syndrome presupposes the existence from birth of an abnormal anatomical communication an accessory pathway (AP), allowing of the possibility of atrioventricular (AV) and/or ventriculoatrial conduction via a route other than the AV node,

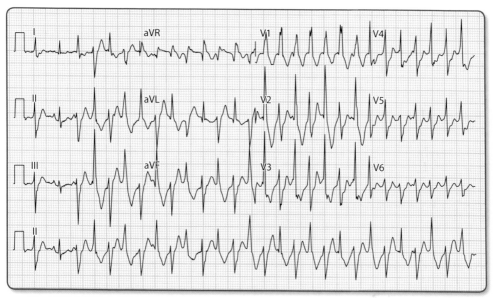

Figure 2.6 Typical catecholaminergic polymorphic ventricular tachycardia (CPVT). The second beat is a sinus beat. This is followed by the onset of typical CPVT. During the VT the frontal plane QRS axis alternates between +135⁰ and −75⁰. The QRS complexes in the precordial leads have alternating morphology, but the two waveforms are not as grossly different as those in the limb leads. ECG courtesy of Dr Simon Modi, Liverpool Heart and Chest Hospital NHS Foundation Trust, Liverpool, UK.

and the His bundle and requires a history of paroxysmal tachycardia. When conduction from atria to ventricles occurs via an AP the typical ECG appearances of ventricular pre-excitation are seen. The finding of ventricular pre-excitation without a history of paroxysmal tachycardia does not justify the use of the term 'WPW syndrome'.

It is well recognised that SCD can occur in the WPW syndrome and that it can be the clinical manifestation of the presence of a previously asymptomatic and/or unrecognised AP. However, many persons (perhaps 50%) with ECG evidence of pre-excitation never develop arrhythmias and, of those with true WPW, only a small minority experience syncope or sudden death.

Prevalence and genetics of pre-excitation and of WPW syndrome

The prevalence of pre-excitation on the 12-lead ECG is thought to be in the region of 0.2% of the population, but the prevalence of the WPW syndrome is substantially less. The prevalence of WPW syndrome in first-degree relatives of those with that condition is thought to be in the region of 2–3 times higher than in the general population. The majority of patients with WPW syndrome have no structural cardiac abnormality (apart from the AP), but some congenital abnormalities are associated with a higher prevalence of WPW syndrome (particularly, Ebstein's anomaly of the tricuspid valve).

The ECG findings (ventricular pre-excitation) in WPW

The ECG findings in ventricular pre-excitation are well known to consist of a short PR interval, a slurring of the initial part of the QRS complex (the Δ wave), broadening of the

QRS complexes and nonspecific ST,T changes secondary to the QRS abnormality. Because of the numerous possible locations (around the AV junction) at which an AP can be found, there are many possible QRS configurations in patients with ventricular pre-excitation. The ECG appearances, therefore, can simulate right or left bundle branch block, right or left ventricular hypertrophy, inferior or anterior infarction or any combination of these. In a given patient, the ECG appearances may vary from those of maximal pre-excitation, to the absence of detectable pre-excitation with any intermediate degree of pre-excitation being possible.

Risk stratification in pre-excitation and in WPW

The majority of patients with ventricular pre-excitation are asymptomatic, the abnormality being discovered on an ECG taken for any of a variety of reasons, and the majority of patients with WPW syndrome have a normal prognosis. The commonest arrhythmia occurring in WPW is atrioventricular re-entrant tachycardia (AVRT). This is typically symptomatic but not life threatening. The second commonest arrhythmia is atrial fibrillation. Atrial fibrillation in WPW syndrome is much commoner than one would anticipate from the background prevalence of structural heart disease, suggesting that either that the episodes of AVRT or the presence of the AP may predispose to this arrhythmia, though the mechanism is not clear.

Atrial fibrillation, and the much less common atrial flutter, do pose a risk of sudden death in those with APs because the AV node is bypassed and very rapid (nondecremental) conduction down the AP(s) is possible, giving rise to ventricular rates of 200–300 per minute (**Figure 2.7**), with the consequent risk of degeneration into VF. The VF risk in atrial fibrillation is highest whenever one or more RR intervals shorter than 250 ms is seen.

The main practical problem relates to the estimation of risk in the asymptomatic subject. It is clear that the later in life that pre-excitation is discovered the lower is the ongoing risk of SCD and that only those patients with rapidly conducting APs appear to be at risk of SCD. When pre-excitation is intermittent or when it suddenly ceases during an exercise test it is

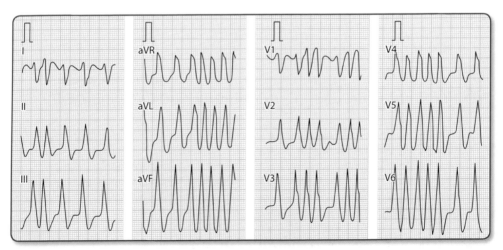

Figure 2.7 Pre-excited atrial fibrillation. Atrial depolarisations are conducted to the ventricles via the rapidly conducting accessory pathway(s) rather than through the more slowly conducting atrioventricular node. The QRS complexes have bizarre shapes which, in this case, tend to be similar in any one lead, the rate is totally irregular and some RR intervals are shorter than 250 ms.

highly unlikely that the AP is rapidly conducting, so ambulatory electrocardiography and exercise electrocardiography do have some value in identifying low-risk cases.

Patients with WPW syndrome who are symptomatically disturbed by episodes of AVRT should be considered for ablation of the AP(s). Ablation is clearly indicated in all those with evidence of pre-excitation and a history of either atrial flutter or atrial fibrillation.

CONGENITAL CORONARY ANOMALIES AND PREMATURE CORONARY DISEASE

Congenital coronary artery anomalies (CAAs) are readily detectable in the paediatric population by transthoracic echocardiography [30], but large-scale screening is not economically feasible. These anomalies are rare, being found in 0.17% of 2388 children and adolescents with anatomically normal hearts referred for echocardiographic assessment (e.g. for murmurs which proved to be innocent, or for functional assessment) [30]. Congenital CAAs are thought to account for about 20% of sudden deaths in American athletes [31]. The possibility of this condition should be considered when young adults experience exertion-related chest discomfort.

Screening processes for coronary risk factors are well studied and readily available. Although the mortality rates from occult coronary disease in the young are very small, the enormous size of this apparently healthy population means that the total annual death rate in this group far exceeds than that from the very small groups with hereditable cardiomyopathies and 'electrical' conditions, even though the latter carry substantially higher death risks. The implication from this is that, in population terms, screening for, and management of, the known coronary risk factors is likely to have a greater impact on total mortality than targeted screening of high noncoronary risk groups.

SCD IN DILATED CARDIOMYOPATHY

About 30% of the overall cardiac mortality in those with dilated cardiomyopathy is via SCD, the remainder of the mortality being mainly from progressive congestive cardiac failure. Of those in class IV heart failure, the majority die from progressive heart failure, with about 20–30% experiencing sudden (but clearly not entirely unexpected) cardiac death. The overall death rates are lower in those with class I or II heart failure but 50–60% of deaths in these groups are sudden [32]. This issue will not be discussed further here since, in the majority of cases, the patient will be known to have a cardiomyopathy and the possibility of sudden death will, therefore, be acknowledged.

SCD IN ATHLETES

Athletes represent a special group in relation to SCD. They are predominantly young and fit and they are repeatedly exposed to the risks of high-level exercise, which can lead to SCD in those with underlying (and usually unsuspected) cardiac abnormalities.

Incidence and aetiology of SCD in athletes

Estimates of the incidence of SCD in athletes vary from 1 in 100,000 per year (US high school and college athletes) to 3 in 100,000 per year (Italian athletes, age range 12–35)

[33]. Italian data suggest that athletes are 2.8 times more likely to experience SCD than nonathletes.

In athletes older than 35, the commonest cause of death is coronary disease. In young athletes, exercise-related death is predominantly cardiac. The commonest cause of exertion-related death in under 35s is HCM. A study of 1866 deaths in young competitive athletes in the United States between 1980 and 2006 [34] showed that 1049 cases (56%) were cardiac deaths, 22% resulted from trauma, 3% were due to commotio cordis (sudden death or cardiac arrest from a precordial blow not giving rise to significant structural injury to the chest wall or to the heart), 8% were of unresolved aetiology and 10% were due to a variety of noncardiac causes. The commonest cardiac cause was HCM (251 cases: 36%, with a further 57 cases being 'possible HCM' at autopsy). The second commonest was congenital CAAs (principally, a coronary artery arising from an inappropriate coronary sinus). The next commonest cause was the group of nonhereditary cardiomyopathy myocarditis and cardiomyopathy followed by the 'electrical' disorders. Within the latter group it was striking that WPW was a rare cause of SCD (14 of the 1049 cases – 1.3%). Non-Whites showed higher risks than Whites in relation to HCM (20% vs. 10%) and CAA (10% vs. 5%) whereas Whites had a higher incidence of SCD from electrical disorders (2% vs. 0.3%).

The athlete's ECG

ECGs taken from athletes frequently show features less commonly seen in ECGs of healthy nonathletes from otherwise similar backgrounds. These features are predominantly training-related changes reflecting both the cardiac rhythm (primarily from increased vagal activity) and physiological left ventricular hypertrophy (with increased QRS voltages). Training-related changes are not known to be associated with increased risk and are potentially reversible with detraining. Some appearances are known to be associated with ethnicity and do not usually carry prognostic significance. Nontraining-related changes (both in relation to rhythm and to morphology) should be regarded as significant (**Table 2.2**).

Screening of athletes

Since high-level, competitive exercise is known to carry a risk of SCD in a selected minority, preparticipation screening is clearly desirable. The more difficult questions relate to the optimal methods, the effectiveness and the cost.

US and European approaches to the screening of athletes

The 36th ACC Bethesda Conference (2005) and the consensus document from the European Society of Cardiology (2005) present many similar recommendations, but the European and American screening strategies differ in one important respect – the use of the ECG. The American screening strategy is confined to the taking of a medical history and the performance of a physical examination. The European strategy (based on extensive experience over many years in Italy) routinely includes a 12-lead ECG. Such a screening process has been in place in the Veneto region of Italy for >30 years, during which time the rate of SCD per 100,000 in athletes fell from 3.6 to 0.4 while that of the unscreened, nonathletic population did not change significantly [33].

Table 2.2 The ECG in athletes*		
Training-related changes	Rhythm	Sinus bradycardia Prolonged PR interval Type 1 second-degree AV block Low atrial rhythm Junctional escape rhythm
	Morphology	Increased QRS voltages Early repolarisation† Partial right bundle branch block (small secondary *r* in V$_1$, QRS duration normal)
Ethnic variations	Morphology	Domed ST elevation with T wave inversion in V$_1$–V$_4$ in Black athletes
Nontraining-related changes	Rhythm	Type 2 second-degree AV block Complete heart block Nonsustained ventricular tachycardia Sustained ventricular tachycardia Atrial fibrillation Atrial flutter
	Morphology	T wave inversion V$_3$–V$_6$ T wave inversion V$_1$–V$_3$ (in whites and without domed ST segments) ST segment depression Pathological Q waves Right or left bundle branch block Long or short QT interval Right ventricular hypertrophy Brugada type 1 pattern Right or left axis deviation (minor factor) Left or right atrial hypertrophy (minor factor)

*Training-related changes and ethnic variations do not, in themselves, give rise to concern. Nontraining-related changes are abnormal and are likely, in varying degree, to be prognostically significant.
†Early repolarisation is noted in up to 9% of the general population, up to 20% of noncompetitive athletes and up to 90% of competitive athletes.

Key points for clinical practice

- CCAs, occult premature coronary disease, inherited cardiomyopathies and 'electrical' syndromes are the major causes of SUCD in young adults.
- Occult coronary disease carries a lower mortality rate than the other categories but the absolute numbers with the latter are very small so their contribution to the population burden of SUCD is low.
- HCM is a common cause of unexpected SUCD in young adults. Patients with this condition need careful evaluation and management. They should avoid high-level, competitive physical activity, beta-blockers should be given when appropriate and an ICD* should be implanted in those with prior cardiac arrest.
- ARVC should be considered in young adults with exertion-related syncope or with precordial T wave changes beyond V$_1$ and V$_2$. Those diagnosed with this condition should be forbidden from taking part in competitive sports. Treatment with beta-blockers may be indicated and those with prior syncope or cardiac arrest should be evaluated for ICD* implantation.

- Patients with LQTS should be assessed and supervised by an expert. They should avoid electrolyte disturbances and QT prolonging drugs. The risks of stress and exercise (LQT1) and of sudden noises or alarms, on a background of rest or sleep (LQT2) should be explained. ICD implantation may be needed in a minority of cases.*

- The majority of patients with sudden death from BrS are asymptomatic before the event. Those with BrS and a prior cardiac arrest require an ICD*. Those with BrS and prior syncope or demonstrated VT should be considered for an ICD*.

- CPVT is a rare condition with a high incidence of SUCD. The resting ECG is usually normal. The condition typically presents with exertion-related bidirectional VT, syncope or SUCD. Competitive exercise should be forbidden and beta-blockers used (unless contraindicated). Patients with cardiac arrest while receiving beta-blockers should be considered for an ICD*.

- The majority of patients with WPW syndrome have a very good prognosis. Those with demonstrated atrial fibrillation or flutter and those with symptomatic atrioventricular re-entrant arrhythmias should be recommended to undergo ablation of the AP(s).

- Screening procedures (including an ECG) should be undertaken for all participating in high-level, competitive sporting activities.

- *ICD implantation has its own acute risks and its own subsequent morbidity. In all cases, the final decision rests on an assessment of the risk–benefit ratio. The current, generally accepted, guide is that ICD insertion is not justifiable unless the anticipated mortality rate for the given condition is ≥1% per annum [35].

REFERENCES

1. Kong MH, Fonarow GC, Peterson ED, et al. Systematic review of the incidence of sudden cardiac death in the United States. J Am Coll Cardiol 2011; 57:794–801.

2A. Myerburg RJ, Castellanos A. Cardiac arrest and sudden cardiac death. In: Mann DL, Zipes DP, Libby P, Bonow RO (eds), Braunwald's heart disease: a textbook of cardiovascular medicine, chapter 39, pages 821-860. Elsevier: Philadelphia, PA, 2015.

2B. Cardiac arrest and sudden cardiac death. Chapter 39. In: Braunwald's heart disease. A textbook of cardiovascular medicine. Mann Dl, Zipes DP, Libby P, et al. (eds). Philadelphia; Elsevier Saunders, 2015:821-860.

3. Papadakis M, Sharma S, Cox S, et al. The magnitude of sudden cardiac death in the young: a death certificate-based review in England and Wales. Europace 2009; 11:1253–1358.

4. Bastiaenen R, Behr EJ. Sudden death and ion channel disease: pathophysiology and implications for management. Heart 2011; 97:1365–1372.

5. Meyer L, Stubbs B, Fahrenbruch C, et al. Incidence, causes, and survival trends from cardiovascular-related sudden cardiac arrest in children and young adults 0 to 35 years of age: a 30-year review. Circulation 2012; 126:1363–1372.

6. van der Werf C, van Langen IM, Wilde AAM. Sudden death in the young. What do we know about it and how to prevent it? Circ Arrhythm Electrophysiol 2010; 3:96–104.

7. Harmon KG, Asif IM, Klossner D, et al. Incidence of sudden cardiac death in national collegiate athletic association athletes. Circulation 2011; 123:1594–1600.

8. Gersh BJ, Maron BJ, Bonow RO, et al. ACCF/AHA guideline for the diagnosis and treatment of hypertrophic cardiomyopathy. J Am Coll Cardiol 2011; 58:2703–2738.

9. Maron BJ, Maron MS, Semsarian C. Genetics of hypertrophic cardiomyopathy after 20 years. J Am Coll Cardiol 2012; 60:705–715.

10. Maron BJ, Casey SA, Hauser RG, et al. Clinical course of hypertrophic cardiomyopathy with survival to advanced age. J Am Coll Cardiol 2002; 42: 882–888.

11. Soraja P, Nishimura RA, Gersh BJ, et al. Outcome of mildly symptomatic or asymptomatic obstructive hypertrophic cardiomyopathy. J Am Coll Cardiol 2009; 54:234–241.

12. Maron BJ and Olivotto I. Chapter 66. In Braunwald's heart disease. A textbook of cardiovascular Medicine. Mann DL, Zipes DP, Libby P, et al. (eds). Philadelphia; Elsevier Saunders, 2015:1574-1588.

13. Konno T, Shimizu M, Ino H, et al. Diagnostic value of abnormal Q waves for identification of preclinical carriers of hypertrophic cardiomyopathy based on a molecular genetic diagnosis. Eur Heart J 2004; 254:246–251.

14. Uberoi A, Stein R, Perez MV, et al. Interpretation of the electrocardiogram of young athletes. Circulation 2011; 124:746–757.

15. McLeod CJ, Ackerman MJ, Nishimura RA, et al. Outcome of patients with hypertrophic cardiomyopathy and a normal electrocardiogram. J Am Coll Cardiol 2009; 54:229–233.

16. Maron BJ, Zipes DP (co-chairs). 36th Bethesda conference: eligibility recommendations for competitive athletes with cardiovascular abnormalities. Circulation 2005; 45:1340–1345.

17. Issa ZF, Miller JM, Zipes DP. Ventricular tachycardia in arrhythmogenic right ventricular cardiomyopathy – dysplasia. In: Josephson ME (ed.), Clinical arrhythmology and electrophysiology: a companion to Braunwald's heart disease, 2nd edn, chapter 29. Philadelphia, PA: Elsevier Saunders, 2012:625–639.

18. James CA, Bhonsale A, Tichnell C, et al. Exercise increases age-related penetrance and arrhythmic risk in arrhythmogenic right ventricular dysplasia/cardiomyopathy-associated desmosomal mutation carriers. J Am Coll Cardiol 2013; 62:1290–1297.

19. Macfarlane PW and Lawrie TDV. In: Macfarlane PW, van Oosterom A, Janse M, et al. (eds), Electrocardiology: Comprehensive Clinical ECG, chapter 1. London: Springer-Verlag, 2010:1-66.

20. Priori SG, Wilde AA, Horie M, et al. HRS/EHRA/APHRS expert consensus statement on the diagnosis and management of patients with inherited primary arrhythmia syndromes. Heart Rhythm 2013; 15:1389–1406.

21. Tester DJ, Ackerman MJ. Postmortem long QT syndrome genetic testing for sudden unexplained death in the young. J Am Coll Cardiol 2007; 49:240–246.

22. Issa ZF, Miller JM, Zipes DP. Ventricular arrhythmias in inherited channelopathies. In: Josephson ME (ed.), Clinical arrhythmology and electrophysiology: a companion to Braunwald's heart disease, 2nd edn, chapter 31. Philadelphia, PA: Elsevier Saunders, 2012.

23. Schwartz PJ. Genetic diseases; the long QT syndrome. In: Saksena S, Camm AJ (eds), Electrophysiological disorders of the heart, chapter 62, Philadelphia, PA: Elsevier Saunders, 2012:875-833.

24. Rowlands DJ, Moore PR. The electrocardiography of the QT interval. Chapter 4, In: Rowlands DJ and Clarke B (Eds). Recent Advances in Cardiology 16. London; JP Medical Limited, 2014:49-67.

25. Goldenberg I, Bradley J, Moss A, et al. Beta-blocker efficiency in high-risk patients with the congenital long-QT syndrome types 1 and 2: implications for patient management. J Cardiovasc Electrophysiol 2010; 21:893–901.

26. Mizusawa Y, Wilde AAM. Brugada syndrome. Circ Arrhythm Electrophysiol 2012; 5:606–616.

27. Antzelevitch c, Brugada P, Borggrefe M, et al. Brugada syndrome: report of the second consensus conference: endorsed by the Heart Rhythm Society and the European Heart Association. Circulation 2005; 111:659–670.

28 Morita H, Kusano KF, Miura D, et al. Fragmented QRS as a marker of conduction abnormality and a predictor of prognosis of Brugada syndrome. Circulation 2008; 118:1697–1704.

29. Napolitano C, Ruan Y, Priori SG. Catecholaminergic Polymorphic Ventricular Tachycardia. Chapter 70. In: Zipes DP, Jalife J (eds), Cardiac electrophysiology, Philadelphia: Elsevier Saunders, 2009:745-751.

30. Davies JA, Cecchin F, Jones TK, et al. Major coronary artery anomalies in a pediatric population: incidence and clinical importance. J Am Coll Cardiol 2001; 37:593–597.

31. Pelliccia A. Congenital coronary artery anomalies in young patients. J Am Coll Cardiol 2001; 37:598–560.

32. Kjekshus J. Arrhythmias and mortality in congestive heart failure. Am J Cardiol 1990; 65:421–481.

33. Corrado D, Basso C, Schiavon M, et al. Pre-participation screening of young competitive athletes for prevention of sudden cardiac death. J Am Coll Cardiol 2008; 52:1981–1989.

34. Maron BJ, Doerer JJ, Hass TS, et al. Sudden deaths in young competitive athletes: analysis of 1866 deaths in the United States, 1980–2006. Circulation 2009; 119:1085–1092.

35. Garratt CJ, Elliott P, Behr E, et al. Heart rhythm UK position on clinical indications for implantable cardioverter defibrillators in adult patients with familial sudden cardiac death syndromes. Europace 2010; 12:1156–1175.

Chapter 3

Out-of-hospital cardiac arrest: survival, immediate and long-term management, and strategies for improvement

Niall O'Keeffe, Mark Forrest

INTRODUCTION

The first reference to resuscitation can be traced back to the Book of Kings in the Old Testament, when Elijah brought a boy back to life using what is effectively described as mouth-to-mouth resuscitation [1]. Many diverse and bizarre techniques for resuscitation have been advocated since then over the years; these include pulling on the tongue and rectal stretching. In 1892, Friedrich Maass reported the first closed chest cardiac massage on a person, but it was not until 1958 that Kouwenhoven and Knickerbocker published a paper outlining its use in clinical practice [2]. The year after the publication of this paper, Safar et al published a paper proposing that the maintenance of a patent airway and intermittent positive pressure ventilation should be used in conjunction with closed chest cardiac massage for optimal outcome [3]. While the technique has subsequently been modified over the years, this paper outlined the basic principles essential to effective resuscitation. They also made the observation that this technique could be taught to nonmedical personnel and could be applied outside the hospital environment. This was essentially the birth of modern cardiopulmonary resuscitation (CPR) as we know it.

It was also around this time that defibrillators were introduced into clinical practice. Dr John McWilliam first described ventricular fibrillation (VF) in 1889, but the initial use of electric shock therapy in resuscitation was aimed at stimulating a physical response from the individual rather than modifying cardiac rhythm. In 1933, Hooker and Kouwenhoven demonstrated that defibrillation could be carried out on a closed chest in dogs. The first successful defibrillation in a patient was carried out by Claude Beck on a 14-year-old boy undergoing thoracic surgery in 1947, and the first successful closed chest defibrillation was reported by Zoll in 1955 [1]. Since then, developments in the technology have resulted

Niall O'Keeffe MB BAO BCh FRCA FICM, Cardiothoracic Anaesthesia and Intensive Care, Manchester Royal Infirmary, Manchester UK

Mark Forrest MB ChB FRCA FICM, Department of Anaesthesia, Manchester Royal Infirmary, Manchester UK. Email: nok@doctors.org.uk (for correspondence)

in the availability of automatic external defibrillatore (AEDs) which, when connected by adhesive paddles to the victim, will analyse the rhythm, advise and shock appropriately. AEDs are designed to be used by nonmedical personnel and can now be found in many public places including supermarkets, bus stations, airports and even hospital waiting rooms (**Figure 3.1**). Seattle has taken this a step further by creating a registry of these devices so that bystanders can be directed to the nearest device when they contact the emergency services to report an arrest.

GUIDELINES

The first guidelines in resuscitation were published in 1966, but at that time wide dissemination to the public was not advocated because of concern about iatrogenic complications [1]. It was not until 1970 that a project in Seattle, which set out to educate the public on the principles and practice of bystander CPR, proved to be very successful, and following that, training of the general public was formally sanctioned in 1974 [1].

Recognition of the fact that an out-of-hospital cardiac arrest (OHCA), if managed promptly and appropriately, is potentially survivable with full recovery has meant that the issue of out-of-hospital arrests and their management has become a major public health topic which now attracts significant investment and resources for both equipment and training. There are a large number of national and international organisations which focus

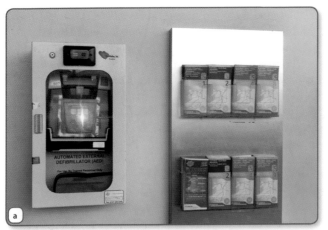
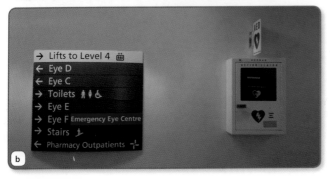

Figure 3.1 Automatic external defibrillators (AED) are increasingly available in the public arena. An AED in a railway station (a) and one in a public area within a hospital (b).

on CPR and whose goals are to deliver a consistent approach to how CPR should be carried out. These include the International Liaison Committee On Resuscitation (ILCOR), the European Resuscitation Council (ERC), the American Heart Association (AHA) and the British Resuscitation Council (BRC).

ILCOR was formed in 1992 and was set up to co-ordinate and provide a forum for discussion of cardiopulmonary and cerebral resuscitation worldwide. ILCOR publishes the Consensus on Resuscitation Science and Treatment Recommendations document. This document is used by various national bodies including the ERC and the BRC to produce their own national guidelines. The first consensus document was published in 2000, and further updates have been published every 5 years. The most recent document was published in 2010 and the next document is scheduled for publication in 2015.

The 'chain of survival' concept was first described in 1991 in a statement from the AHA and has since then been almost uniformly adopted by the various national and international organisations [4]. It sets out to communicate the sequence of events which should occur as rapidly as possible to optimise survival. It was subsequently revised in 2005 to reflect the importance of recognising impending arrest before it occurs and the importance of appropriate post resuscitation care (**Figure 3.2**) [5].

A number of mechanical devices have been developed for external chest compression, but to date none of these has been shown to improve outcomes, although it has to be recognised that there are many difficulties around research studies in these population groups. One major difficulty in comparing data has been in ensuring that like is compared with like because of the complex background, widely varying nomenclature and lack of standard definitions.

In an attempt to address this issue, a major international multidisciplinary meeting was convened in 1991 at Utstein Abbey in Norway and criteria were published to establish uniform terms and definitions for out-of-hospital resuscitation. These are now referred to as the Utstein style in a similar way that the Vancouver style defines technical requirements for written submissions to medical journals [6]. The meeting produced standardised resuscitation terminology, most of which is still in use today. It introduced the concepts of basic life support (BLS) and advanced life support, and also produced a template for reporting data from resuscitation studies to facilitate comparability. It stratifies arrests initially by the status of the witness (no witness, untrained or trained responder) and then by initial rhythm. Utstein survival refers to hospital survival of those cardiac patients whose arrest was witnessed by a bystander and whose initial rhythm was VF or pulseless ventricular tachycardia (VT), as these patients are most likely to respond to therapy and, therefore, most likely to survive. The template was revised and simplified in 2004 with the aim of improving data definition and allowing more accurate completion [7].

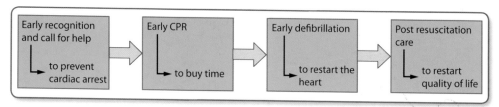

Figure 3.2 The 'chain of survival' concept was introduced in 1991 and updated in 2005 [5].

There is ongoing discussion over the role of respiratory support in out-of-hospital arrests. Certainly, the ultimate goal is an airway protected by a cuffed endotracheal tube to protect the lungs from aspiration and also allow optimal ventilation, but this must not be at the expense of significant interruption in cardiac compressions. While intubation provides airway protection superior to that provided by other airway devices, loss of cardiac output due to interruption of cardiac massage while the endotracheal tube is being placed may contribute to hypoxic brain injury, and unrecognised misplacement of the endotracheal tube in the oesophagus may mean loss of oxygenation completely. There is evidence that, with untrained bystanders receiving telephone instructions, outcomes may be better with cardiac compressions alone rather than with combined cardiac compressions and attempted artificial ventilation [8]. Even intubation by trained medical staff can lead to significant interruption to chest compressions, and there are a number of supraglottic airway devices now available which are easy to place and provide a good airway, and although they do not protect against aspiration they are increasingly being used for both OHCA and in-hospital arrests (**Figure 3.3**).

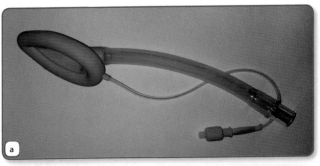
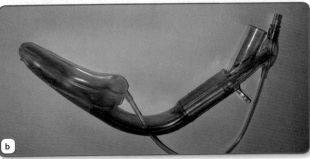
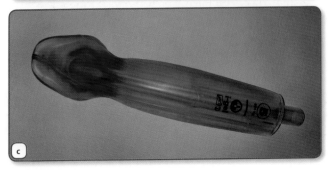

Figure 3.3 There are a number of airway devices now available which are relatively easy to place and in most cases provide a good airway. (a) Original laryngeal mask airway, (b) laryngeal mask supreme (this has two lumens and in theory the second lumen would direct regurgitated stomach contents away from the larynx) and (c) I-gel (this has a solid gel cuff).

However, there are a number of circumstances where combined cardiac massage and respiratory support have been shown to be beneficial. These include young patients, arrest of noncardiac origin, delay before CPR initiation and prolonged arrest of cardiac origin [9].

The most recent recommendations of ILCOR, which are cascaded down through the national resuscitation councils, reflect some of this research [9]. A key change identified in the 2010 document was a shift from the time honoured airway, breathing and circulation (ABC) of resuscitation to compressions/circulation, airway, breathing (CAB) to reflect the recognised importance of early chest compressions, which can be particularly important in a witnessed arrest [9]. Bystanders who are not trained should provide compressions only, while those with BLS training should also provide ventilations with a compression–ventilation ratio of 30:2. Emergency medical services (EMS) dispatchers who are providing telephone support to untrained bystanders should advise CPR with compressions only. The other key recommended change is that CPR should be commenced if the victim is unresponsive and not breathing properly, without checking for a pulse [9].

Although all current guidelines include the use of adrenaline, more recently its use has been questioned because of its effect on microcirculation, potentially resulting in cerebral ischaemia. Paramedic 2 – the Adrenaline Trial – is a controversial trial involving five ambulance services in the United Kingdom in which patients suffering from OHCA are randomised to receive adrenaline, where indicated, or placebo, obviously without their consent to be included in the study. While this study has provoked ethical debate over the inclusion of patients without their consent, it started recruiting in December 2014.

HOSPITAL MANAGEMENT OF OHCA

Following admission to hospital the immediate care involves assessment and stabilisation. If the patient is unconscious, the airway should be protected with a cuffed endotracheal tube and haemodynamic stability achieved with inotropes and mechanical-assist devices, if necessary. A trigger for the arrest should be identified where possible.

Out-of-hospital arrests occur from many causes, but the majority have a cardiac cause, most commonly ischaemic heart disease. Other cardiac causes include cardiomyopathy and valvular disease, and rarer causes include inherited conditions such as long QT syndrome (estimated incidence 0.05%), short QT syndrome (estimated incidence 0.02%) or Brugada syndrome (estimated incidence 0.01–0.05%) [10]. Syncope is an independent risk factor for sudden death.

Return of spontaneous circulation (ROSC) following cardiac arrest is often associated with both ischaemic and reperfusion injuries in multiple areas throughout the body, affecting not only the heart but also multiple organs including the brain, the lungs and the kidneys. This has been referred to as the postcardiac arrest syndrome [11]. It is often complicated by the original cause of the arrest, which may remain a threat and may need addressing. A key element of optimisation is close and comprehensive monitoring and attention to detail. If there is evidence of myocardial ischaemia, then primary percutaneous intervention (PCI) should be considered. All patients with impaired conscious levels or shock will require critical care for an undefined period ranging from days to several weeks. Early critical care management should focus on treating cardiovascular instability, measures aimed at improving neurological outcome and treating any other complications of OHCA such as aspiration. In the intermediate and longer term, the management of cardiovascular conditions, notably heart failure, and neurological complications, including seizures and impaired cognitive function, come to the fore.

Cardiovascular management

The incidence of circulatory impairment following spontaneous restoration of circulation or primary PCI is possibly as high as two-thirds, compared with 10% for all acute myocardial infarction (AMI) admissions. The mortality in those patients with cardiogenic shock who reach the intensive care unit (ICU) after OHCA is reported at over 20% [12]. The aetiology is often multifactorial, including hypovolaemia, cardiogenic shock secondary either to myocardial infarction with stunning or arrhythmia, and vasodilatation as part of a systemic inflammatory response syndrome (SIRS). A package of measures including fluid resuscitation, inotropes, vasopressors, antiarrhythmics and mechanical support for those with refractory hypotension seems intuitive and is successful for many patients. One paper has suggested that norepinephrine, while offering no benefit in terms of survival when compared with dopamine, is associated with fewer untoward events and might, therefore, be preferable [13]. Levosimendan, a calcium channel sensitiser, has been shown to reduce mortality from cardiogenic shock when compared with both dobutamine and enoximone [14,15]. However, these studies are small, often with confounding factors, and a recent Cochrane review of the use of inotropes in cardiogenic shock concluded that there were no robust and convincing data to support a distinct inotropic or vasodilator drug-based therapy as a superior solution to reduce mortality in haemodynamically unstable patients with cardiogenic shock or low cardiac output complicating AMI [16]. This is reflected in the 2010 AHA postcardiac arrest guidelines [17]. Having said that, the combination of a phosphodiesterase inhibitor, e.g. enoximone or milrinone, and norepinephrine with intra-aortic balloon counterpulsation therapy (IABP), if necessary, is a commonly used combination. While IABP therapy is used in many centres, the base of evidence is poor. The IABP-SHOCK II trial concluded that use of IABP in cardiogenic shock did not reduce all that cause mortality at 12 months [18]. Ventricular-assist devices and venous–arterial extra-corporeal membrane oxygenation have been used extensively in the management of refractory cardiogenic shock with reports of positive outcomes following cardiac arrest, although there are currently no controlled trials looking at the efficacy of this. It is also important, when instituting advanced mechanical support, that consideration is given to the exit strategy. It might be that there is a degree of myocardial stunning with the possibility of improvement in ventricular contractility which would allow weaning from the assist device within a short time frame. Some assist devices are suitable to use as a bridge to heart transplantation, while others are less so. However, regardless of the suitability of a given device, institution of mechanical support as a bridge in circumstances where the neurological outcome is uncertain is at best a complex decision which requires careful consideration before implementation.

Whatever the cause of haemodynamic instability, echocardiography is important for guiding therapy, and haemodynamic instability is a Level 1 indication for echocardiography. Image quality is superior with transoesophageal echocardiography (TOE) when patients' lungs are being ventilated, and this should be used if possible. Hypovolaemia, poor myocardial contractility and vasodilatation are all readily diagnosed using TOE. It does not require a high level of expertise to make the diagnoses and there is a high level of reporting consistency. TOE can also be used to assess the response to therapies and their weaning.

Arrhythmias following ROSC after cardiac arrest are common, with an incidence of VF or VT of around 5%, while patients remain in hospital. BRC guidelines suggest the use of amiodarone for the management of VT with a pulse, and cardioversion for pulseless VT, VF or VT associated with signs of poor cardiac output [19].

There is some evidence that beta-blockers can reduce recurrent VF and improve short- and long-term survival [17]. In patients where inotropic or vasopressor support is still required, there may be a role for rate control with ivabradine. The use of steroids remains controversial, but they may have a role particularly where vasopressor requirements are high.

All patients following OHCA should be considered for implantable cardioverter defibrillator therapy prior to leaving hospital.

Neurological considerations

Following OHCA many patients remain comatose, defined as a lack of meaningful response to verbal commands, on admission to hospital despite ROSC and management should be directed at reducing the deleterious effects of the probable cerebral hypoxia. Two studies published at similar times in 2002 demonstrated that the use of mild hypothermia, i.e. cooling to a core temperature between 32°C and 34°C, was associated with a significant increase in the number of patients discharged from hospital with good neurological outcome [20,21]. These studies looked at patients where the arrest rhythm was VF. There are no randomised studies looking at the benefits of cooling where the rhythm was something other than VF, although studies have shown a benefit against historical controls when looking at survivors of OHCA with any rhythm [22].

Current AHA guidelines and a Cochrane review would favour the use of mild hypothermia (32–34°C) in all survivors of OHCA [17]. There is no evidence of benefit in cooling to lower temperatures, and temperatures below 32°C are associated with a higher incidence of complications including arrhythmias, coagulopathy and gastric stasis that, in turn, can prevent feeding and increase the incidence of ventilator associated pneumonia. A more recent study has shown that the same neurological outcome is seen with cooling to just 36°C, and it is possible that the prevention of the hyperthermia associated with an inflammatory response is the important therapeutic goal rather than hypothermia per se [23].

The effect of the timing of induced hypothermia is unclear. Intuitively, one would feel that cooling as early as possible would show the greatest benefit. This is backed up by animal studies. However, in humans, studies suggest that hypothermia initiated at 2 h post-ROSC and at 8 h post-ROSC show similar neurological outcomes. Experience would suggest that following OHCA passive cooling occurs to such an extent that patients are often at 35°C or below by the time they reach the ICU. With regard to the duration of hypothermia, most authorities would suggest at least 12 h, while 24 h is the norm [17]. There are no studies looking at hypothermia for periods longer than 24 h in this setting. There are several methods in use for inducing hypothermia including ice packs, infusion of cold fluids and forced air cooling.

Hyperglycaemia is associated with a worsened neurological outcome, but tight glycaemic control is associated with an increased incidence of severe hypoglycaemia that is also likely to worsen neurological outcome. A moderate glycaemic control strategy aiming for blood sugars in the range 8–10 mmol/L is recommended [17].

Hyperventilation, aimed at reducing the arterial pCO_2, has been used in traumatic head injury to reduce cerebral blood flow and thereby intracranial pressure, but there is no place for such a strategy in global ischaemic brain injury where on the contrary reducing cerebral blood flow is likely to worsen the outcome. Ventilatory strategy should in general aim for normocapnia.

Sedation

Most patients admitted to the ICU following OHCA will require sedation at least for a short period to facilitate mechanical ventilation and to reduce shivering during induced hypothermia. In general, this sedation should be as light as circumstances allow so that early neurological assessment can be made once sedation is discontinued. There is no evidence that choice of sedation makes any difference to outcome, so the choice should be made with pharmacokinetic profiles in mind. The ideal drug would have high clearance and a low volume of distribution. Both remifentanil and propofol fit this profile. Benzodiazepines such as midazolam should probably be avoided as they have a longer half-life and have been implicated as a potential cause of delirium.

Respiratory support

Many patients will require intubation and ventilation following ROSC after OHCA. A comatose condition mandates intubation of the trachea to protect the airway from soiling and ventilation of the lungs is likely to be required while the patient is cooled and sedated.

It is not uncommon to see lung pathology following OHCA, most commonly either pulmonary oedema secondary to left ventricular failure or SIRS or infection particularly following aspiration of gastric contents. Specific treatment will depend on the cause. The ventilatory strategy will be the same as for other ICU patients; a lung protective strategy with high positive end-expiratory pressure, low tidal volumes and low inspiratory pressures. Oxygen therapy should be titrated to achieve normal partial pressures of oxygen in arterial blood. There is evidence that hyperoxygenation can worsen neurological outcome and should be avoided. Oxygen-free radicals have been implicated in cellular toxicity in acute illness, and production of these may be increased with raised oxygen levels. There is growing concern about how oxygen is used in AMI, with very little evidence to support its use and postcardiac-arrest evidence that hyperoxia increases mortality in patients admitted to the ICU [24]. It seems prudent based on current evidence to titrate oxygen administration to achieve normal arterial oxygen levels. ILCOR has advocated aiming for peripheral saturations 94–96% [11].

Intermediate, long-term care and prognostication

Following cooling and slow rewarming, sedation should be discontinued as soon as possible to allow early neurological assessment. Patients fall into two categories on emerging from sedation: those who wake up with essentially normal neurological function and those who exhibit signs of significant neurological impairment.

For those who do not wake up quickly, the differential diagnosis is delayed clearance of any sedative agent used, neurological damage, or, rarely, metabolic derangement. Clearance of sedative agents will depend on their time-sensitive half-life, which, in turn, depends to a certain extent on the mechanism of clearance, volume of distribution and the duration of sedation. For example, remifentanil has a very small volume of distribution and high esterase-based clearance and wears off rapidly. The time taken for it to be cleared is relatively independent of its duration of use. Propofol, on the other hand, is highly lipid soluble and the time to wakening will depend significantly on its duration of use. Increasing age may also affect its clearance. It is metabolised in the liver to inactive metabolites and so is not affected by renal failure. This is in contrast to midazolam which is metabolised to active metabolites that are renally excreted so its duration of action will be affected by renal failure. In general terms, patients sedated with propofol would be expected to be awake within 48 h of its cessation, and where that is not the case other causes for coma should be sought.

Seizure activity is common (10–35%) and is often subclinical. Early electroencephalography (EEG) is important to detect seizure activity [26]. It is generally considered important to stop seizure activity to prevent further cerebral damage and to remove the postictal state as a cause of coma. Phenytoin, valproate, levetiracetam , clonazepam and midazolam are all used regularly, with choice depending on experience and personal preference. It is clear, however, that seizure activity following OHCA is a very poor prognostic sign with a 30-day mortality of between 80 and 100% and almost no good neurological recovery [25,26]. There is currently no evidence that treating seizures improves outcome [27].

Burst suppression is also often seen on EEG post OHCA. This can be confused with the cerebral effects of sedation. Once it is clear that sedative agents are not the cause, however, the outcome is again very poor.

Computerised tomography (CT) of the brain is regularly requested though sensitivity and specificity are not as high as for EEG. While the CT appearances of hypoxic brain injury, including loss of grey/white matter differentiation are well recognised, CT scans are often normal and can rarely show other pathology such as focal cerebrovascular ischaemia or subarachnoid haemorrhage.

Predicting neurological outcome following OHCA can be extremely difficult. Increased time to ROSC and age are both associated with worse outcome, while a shockable presenting rhythm and immediate bystander CPR are associated with better neurological outcome [28,29]. Experience suggests that progression from similar initial neurological pictures can be highly inconsistent and attempts to prognosticate early in the post arrest period are fraught with difficulty.

The degree of neurological recovery encompasses the entire spectrum from normal neurology through to persistent coma. Experience suggests that those who make a good neurological recovery tend to recover early and rapidly, although this is not always the case. Neurological recovery is assessed using the Cerebral Performance Category (CPC) scale which is a widely used five-point scale ranging from normal neurology to persistent coma (Table 3.1). This categorisation is useful for delineating prognosis. Data from Seattle showed that, of nearly 1000 patients resuscitated following OHCA and surviving to discharge, 85% were in CPC 1 or 2. Relative risk of 1-year survival compared with CPC 1 was 0.61 for CPC 2, 0.43 for CPC 3 and 0.1 for CPC 4 [30]. Those who remain in a comatose state 4 weeks after ROSC can be referred to as persistent coma. Improvement after this time in those with anoxic brain injury is highly unlikely. Most of these patients will die within 6 months, although survival may occasionally be for years. Further care will be tailored to need but may include intensive physiotherapy, occupational therapy and rehabilitation. With this sort of care there is some evidence that those surviving to discharge with less than category 1 CPC can make further neurological recovery, although quality of life may be poor in the long term and worse than that of other patients following prolonged critical illness [31]. Pathways for the care of these patients are often underdeveloped and

Table 3.1 Cerebral Performance Categories scale which is used to assess neurological outcome following cardiac arrest [37]

Cerebral Performance Category scale	Neurological outcomes
1. Good cerebral performance	Conscious, alert, able to work and lead a normal life. May have minor psychological or neurologic deficits (mild dysphasia, nonincapacitating hemiparesis, or minor cranial nerve abnormalities)
2. Moderate cerebral disability	Conscious; sufficient cerebral function for part-time work in sheltered environment or independent activities of daily life (dress, travel by public transportation, food preparation). May have hemiplegia, seizures, ataxia, dysarthria, dysphasia or permanent memory or mental changes
3. Severe cerebral disability	Conscious; dependent on others for daily support (in an institution or at home with exceptional family effort). Has at least limited cognition. This category includes a wide range of cerebral abnormalities, from patients who are ambulatory but have severe memory disturbances or dementia precluding independent existence to those who are paralysed and can communicate only with their eyes, as in the locked-in syndrome
4. Coma/vegetative state	Unconscious, unaware of surroundings, no cognition. No verbal or psychological interaction with environment
5. Brain death	Certified brain dead or dead by traditional criteria

under-resourced. If it is established that the long-term prognosis is very poor and further treatment futile, then these patients may be considered for organ donation [11].

OVERALL OUTCOME OF OHCA

The latest figures on survival following nontraumatic OHCA attended by the EMS in the United States were published in January 2014 and are extrapolated from an ongoing registry from the Resuscitation Outcomes Consortium, which is a clinical trial network in North America focusing on prehospital cardiopulmonary arrest and severe traumatic injury [10]. Data are collected and entered in the registry based on assessments made by the EMS [10]. These data suggest that around 424,000 people suffer an OHCA each year in the United States. Around 60% of these patients receive treatment from the EMS, and of these 23% had an initial rhythm of either VF or VT. Prior heart disease was a major risk factor and the incidence is higher among Blacks and Hispanics than among Caucasians. A family history of cardiac arrest in a close relative (parent, sibling or offspring) is associated with a twofold increase in risk.

In 2011, survival to discharge in patients suffering from OHCA treated by the EMS with any recorded initial rhythm was 10.4% overall, 10.7% (95% CI, 9.7–11.2%) for adults and 5.4% (95% CI, 2.4–8.4%) for children. Survival after bystander witnessed VF is 31.7% (95% CI, 28.2–35.1%) for adults, and 26.7% (95% CI, 4.3–49.0%) for children [10].

The mortality of patients who survived to hospital admission was recorded in the United States over the period 2001–2009 using the National Inpatient Sample, a database representing 20% of all nonfederal and nonrehabilitation hospital admissions in the United States [34]. The mean number of admissions following OHCA studied per year was 132,318.

The mortality decreased year on year from 69.6% in 2001 to 57.8% in 2009. Multivariate analysis showed earlier year of admission to be an independent predictor of mortality (P <0.001) [32]. Another retrospective cohort study published in 2012 looked at angioplasty and therapeutic hypothermia. For patients who survive to hospital, 5-year survival is better for those who received angioplasty compared with those who did not (77.5% vs. 60%) [33].

There is increasing focus on patients who have an out-of-hospital arrest when engaging in sporting activities. Kim et al looked at the incidence and outcome of cardiac arrests associated with marathons and half-marathons between 2000 and 2010 [34]. Of 10.9 million runners, 59 suffered a cardiac arrest, an incidence of 0.54 per 100,000 participants, which is low when compared with the general population [34]. The average age was 42±13 years. The probable cause of arrest was available in 31 of the 59, and the commonest cause was hypertrophic cardiomyopathy. Mortality was 42/59 (71%) and survivors were older than nonsurvivors (mean age survivors 49 ± 10 years vs. nonsurvivors 39 ± 9 years) [34].

Seattle has for a long time been a leader in community-based resuscitation and the most recent data from their 2013 annual report states that for bystander witnessed VF survival to hospital discharge is 57%, and the survival rate from all cardiac arrests is 22% [35]. This shows what can be achieved with an absolute commitment to public engagement and education, and the use of novel initiatives such as equipping police with AEDs and identifying them as primary responders as part of the EMS. Other public initiatives in Seattle include training all secondary school students in CPR and showing them how to use an AED by incorporating it into the state's high school curricula. There are an increasing number of AEDs, and in Washington State all AEDs must be registered, which means that despatchers can direct bystanders to the nearest AED while they are waiting for the emergency services to arrive. Seattle also leads on the training of telephone despatchers, not just to liaise with the emergency services but also to talk bystanders through CPR while awaiting the arrival of the emergency services, thereby improving outcome [36]. Outcome figures for Seattle are compared with London and the United States as a whole in **Table 3.2** and demonstrate what can be achieved with a comprehensive approach.

Immense progress has been made involving the public in initiating resuscitation for OHCA, and current evidence suggests there is still potential for further improvement through better education, identification of resuscitation equipment in public areas and comprehensive emergency service networks.

Table 3.2 Survival following OHCA*						
Outcomes	USA 2011		London 2012/2013		Seattle 2012	
	Total	Survival (%)	Total	Survival (%)	Total	Survival (%)
EMS treated	211,000	10.4	3803	9.3	1134	22
EMS treated/shockable rhythm	42,000	28.3			303	47
Bystander witnessed/shockable rhythm	24,000	31.7	556	28.4	193	57

*This table shows latest numbers and outcome variables for the various categories of out-of-hospital cardiac arrest for the United States as a whole, and also for the cities of Seattle in the United States and London in the United Kingdom. EMS, emergency medical services.

Key points for clinical practice

- The ABC approach to resuscitation has been changed to CAB to reflect the importance of external cardiac compressions.

- In the early stages maintaining cardiac output using cardiac compressions is more important than airway management.

- Current guidelines advise that, if a collapsed patient is unresponsive and not breathing properly, CPR should be started without checking for a pulse.

- Early angioplasty is associated with better long-term outcomes.

- Early ICU management is aimed at haemodynamic stabilisation and optimising neurological outcome.

- There is no convincing evidence to support any particular cardiovascular support protocol.

- Cooling to just below 36°C is as effective as moderate hypothermia (32–34°C).

- Long-term neurological outcome can be very difficult to predict in the early stages, particularly in the younger patient.

- Seizure activity is associated with a very poor prognosis even if seizures are controlled.

- The best results worldwide would suggest that of those reaching hospital alive after OHCA 85% can recover to CPC 1. This depends on all aspects of care from the moment of arrest.

REFERENCES

1. Cooper JA, Cooper JD, Cooper JM. Cardiopulmonary resuscitation: history, current practice and future direction. Circulation 2006; 114:2839–2849.
2. Kouwenhoven WB, Jude JR, Knickerbocker GG. Closed chest cardiac massage. JAMA 1960; 173:1064–1067.
3. Safar P, Brown TC, Holtey WJ, Wilder RJ. Ventilation and circulation with closed chest cardiac massage in man. JAMA 1961; 176:574–576.
4. Cummins RO, Ornato WH, Thies WH, Pepe PE. Improving survival from cardiac arrest: the "chain of survival" concept. A statement for health professionals from the Advanced Cardiac Life Support Subcommittee and the Emergency Cardiac Care Committee, American Heart Association. Circulation 1991; 83:1832–1847.
5. Nolan JP, Soar J, Eikeland H. The chain of survival. Resuscitation 2006; 71:270–271.
6. Cummins RO, Chamberlain DA, Abramson NS, et al. Recommended guidelines for uniform reporting of data from out-of-hospital cardiac arrest: the Utstein Style. A statement for health professionals from a task force of the American Heart Association, the European Resuscitation Council, the Heart and Stroke Foundation of Canada, and the Australian Resuscitation Council. Circulation 1991; 84:960–975.
7. Jacobs I, Nadkarni V, Bahr J, et al (The ILCOR Task Force on Cardiac Arrest and Cardiopulmonary Resuscitation Outcomes). Cardiac arrest and cardiopulmonary resuscitation outcome reports: update and simplification of the Utstein templates for resuscitation registries. A statement for healthcare professionals from a task force of the International Liaison Committee on Resuscitation (American Heart Association, New Zealand Resuscitation Council, Heart and Stroke Foundation of Canada, InterAmerican Heart Foundation, Resuscitation Councils of South Africa). Circulation 2004; 110:3385–3397.
8. Dumas F, Rea TD, Fahrenbruch C, et al. Chest compression alone cardiopulmonary resuscitation is associated with better long-term survival compared with standard cardiopulmonary resuscitation. Circulation 2013; 127:435–441.
9. Nolan JP, Hazinski MF, Billi JE. Part 1: executive summary: 2010 International Consensus on Cardiopulmonary Resuscitation and Emergency Cardiovascular Care Science With treatment Recommendations. Resuscitation 2010; 815:e1–e25.
10. Go AS, Mozaffarian D, Roger VL, et al. Heart disease and stoke statistics – 2014 update: a report from the American Heart Association. Circulation 2014; 129:e28–e292.
11. Neumar RW, Nolan JP, Adrie C, et al. Post-cardiac arrest syndrome: epidemiology, pathophysiology, treatment, and prognostication. A consensus statement from the International Liaison Committee

on Resuscitation (American Heart Association, Australian and New Zealand Council on Resuscitation, European Resuscitation Council, Heart and Stroke Foundation of Canada, InterAmerican Heart Foundation, Resuscitation Council of Asia, and the Resuscitation Council of Southern Africa); the American Heart Association Emergency Cardiovascular Care Committee; the Council on Cardiovascular Surgery and Anesthesia; the Council on Cardiopulmonary, Perioperatieve, and Critical Care; the Council on Clinical Cardiology; and the Stroke Council. Circulation 2008; 118:2452–2483.

12. Lemaile V, Dumas F, Mongardon N, et al. Intensive care unit mortality after cardiac arrest: the relative contribution of shock and brain injury in a large cohort. Intensive Care Med 2013; 39:1972–1980.

13. De Backer D, Biston P, Devriendt J, et al. Comparison of dopamine and norepinephrine in the treatment of shock. N Engl J Med 2010; 362:779–789.

14. Landoni G, Biondi-Zoccai G, Greco M, et al. Effects of levosimendan on mortality and hospitalization. A meta-analysis of randomized controlled studies. Crit Care Med 2012; 40:634–646.

15. Fuhrmann J, Schmeisser A, Schulz M, et al. Levosimendan is superior to enoximone in refractory cardiogenic shock complicating acute myocardial infarction. Crit Care Med 2008; 36:2257–2266.

16. Unverzagt S, Wachsmuth L, Hirsch K, et al. Inotropic agents and vasodilator strategies for acute myocardial infarction complicated by cardiogenic shock or low cardiac output syndrome. Cochrane Database Syst Rev 2014 Jan 2; 1:CD009669.

17. Peberdy MA, Callaway CW, Neumar RW, et al. Part 9: post-cardiac arrest care: 2010 American Heart Association Guidelines for Cardiopulmonary Resuscitation and Emergency Cardiovascular Care. Circulation 2010; 122:S768–S786.

18. Holger T, Zeymer U, Neumann F, et al. Intra-aortic balloon counterpulsation in acute myocardial infarction complicated by cardiogenic shock (IABP-SHOCK II): final 12 month results of a randomised, open-label trial. Lancet 2013; 382:1638–1645.

19. Deakin C, Nolan J, Perkins Glockey A. Adult Advanced Life Support. Resuscitation Council (UK) Guidelines 2010. London, UK: Resuscitation Council, 2010. www.resus.org.uk.

20. Holzer M, The Hypothermia After Cardiac Arrest Study Group. Mild therapeutic hypothermia to improve the neurological outcome after cardiac arrest. N Engl J Med 2002; 346:549–556.

21. Bernard SA, Gray TW, Buist MD, et al. Treatment of comatose survivors of out of hospital cardiac arrest with induced hypothermia. N Engl J Med 2002; 346:557–563.

22. Sunde K, Pytte M, Jacobsen D, et al. Implementation of a standard treatment protocol for post resuscitation care after out of hospital cardiac arrest. Resuscitation 2007; 73:29–39.

23. Nielsen N, Wettersley J, Cronberg T, et al. Targeted temperature management at 33°C versus 36°C after cardiac arrest. N Engl J Med 2013; 369:2197–2206.

24. Kilgannon JH, Jones AE, Shapiro NI, et al. Association between arterial hypoxaemia following resuscitation from cardiac arrest and in-patient mortality. JAMA 2010; 303:2165–2171.

25. Sadaka F, Doerr D, Hindia J, et al. Continuous electroencephalogram in comatose postcardiac arrest syndrome patients treated with therapeutic hypothermia: outcome prediction study. J Intensive Care Med 2014; doi: 0885066613517214 (Epub ahead of print).

26. Knight W, Hart K, Opeolu M, et al. The incidence of seizures in patients undergoing therapeutic hypothermia after resuscitation from cardiac arrest. Epilepsy Res 2013; 106:396–402.

27. Hofmeijer J, Tjepkema-Cloostermans M, Blans M, et al. Unstandardized treatment of electroencephalographic status epilepticus does not improve outcome of comatose patients after cardiac arrest. Front Neurol 2014; 5: 1–8.

28. Oddo M, Ribordy V, Feihl F, et al. Early predictors of outcome in comatose survivors of ventricular fibrillation and non-ventricular fibrillation cardiac arrest treated with hypothermia: a prospective study. Crit Care Med 2008; 36:2296–301.

29. Terman S, Hume B, Meurer W, Silbergleit R. Impact of presenting rhythm on short- and long-term neurologic outcome in comatose survivors of cardiac arrest treated with therapeutic hypothermia. Crit Care Med 2014; 42:2225–2234.

30. Phelps R, Dumas F, Maynard C, Silver J, Rea T. Cerebral performance category and long-term prognosis following out-of-hospital cardiac arrest. Crit Care Med 2013; 41:1252–1257.

31. Lim C, Verfaellie M, Schnyer D, Lafleche G, AlexanderM. Recovery, long-term cognitive outcome and quality of life following out-of-hospital cardiac arrest. J Rehabil Med 2014; 46:691–697.

32. Fugate JE, Brinjiki W, Mandrekar JN, et al. Post-cardiac arrest mortality is declining: a study of the US National Inpatient Sample 2001 to 2009. Circulation 2012; 126:546–550.

33. Dumas F, White L, Stubbs BA, et al. Long term prognosis following resuscitation from out of hospital cardiac arrest: role of percutaneous coronary intervention and therapeutic hypothermia. J Am Coll Cardiol 2012; 60:21–27.

34. Kim JH, Malhotra R, Chiampas G, et al. Cardiac arrest during long-distance running races. N Engl J Med 2012; 366:130–140.

35. Chatalas H, Plorde M (eds). Public Health - Seattle & King County. Division of Emergency Medical Services. 2014 Annual Report. Seattle: EMS Division, 2014.

36. White L, Rogers J, Bloomingdale M, et al. Dispatcher-assisted cardiopulmonary resuscitation: risks for patients not in cardiac arrest. Circulation 2010; 121:91–97.

37. Ajam K, Gold LS, Beck SS, et al. Reliability of the Cerebral Performance Category to classify neurological status among survivors of ventricular fibrillation arrest: a cohort study. Scand J Trauma Resusc Emerg Med 2011; 19:38.

Chapter 4

Cardiac biomarkers and risk stratification

Richard Body

INTRODUCTION AND SCOPE

Biomarkers play an essential role in the diagnosis and risk stratification of patients with suspected and confirmed acute coronary syndromes. Biomarkers may have additional applications outside of the acute coronary syndromes, for example in patients with heart failure, transient loss of consciousness or for predicting risk in apparently healthy individuals. There may be clinical applications for biomarkers in congenital heart disease, valvular heart disease, atrial fibrillation and stable angina. This chapter will address the role of biomarkers in the risk stratification and diagnosis of acute coronary syndromes.

A BRIEF HISTORY OF CARDIAC BIOMARKERS

Cardiac biomarkers have been used for the diagnosis of acute myocardial infarction (AMI) since the 1950s. Before the advent of cardiac troponin, AMI could be diagnosed on the basis of a characteristic release pattern of three cardiac enzymes: creatine kinase (CK), lactate dehydrogenase (LDH) and alanine aminotransferase (ALT). The observation of an early rise and fall of CK levels with later rises in serum levels of ALT and LDH was consistent with the diagnosis of AMI. Unfortunately, the biomarkers in use at that time were neither sensitive nor specific for AMI. CK levels will rise following skeletal muscle injury, whereas ALT and LDH levels will rise following liver injury and ALT is also found in bone. A further, significant limitation of this biomarker combination is that it took 72 hours before the diagnosis of AMI could be excluded or 'ruled out', which required a prolonged hospital admission for patients.

The development of assays for the more cardiac-specific MB fraction of CK (CK-MB) promised to improve matters further, although, when used alone, CK-MB still has imperfect sensitivity and specificity for the diagnosis of AMI. The advent of assays for cardiac troponin, however, made it possible to 'rule out' the possibility of AMI as early as 12 hours after a patient's symptoms developed and enabled the detection of myocardial injury with unprecedented sensitivity and specificity. This led to its incorporation into the World Health Organization definition of AMI by the year 2000, which stipulated that a rise and fall of either troponin or CK-MB was required to make the diagnosis except when pathologic findings were available [1].

Richard Body MB ChB MRCSEd (A&E) FCEM PhD, Emergency Department, Manchester Royal Infirmary, Manchester, UK. Email: richard.body@manchester.ac.uk (for correspondence)

Since then, assays for cardiac troponin have improved progressively such that the more recent universal definition of myocardial infarction gives cardiac troponin the central role in the diagnosis of AMI. In summary, the universal definition of myocardial infarction from 2012 requires the following: detection of a rise and/or fall of cardiac troponin with at least one level above the 99th percentile upper reference limit, together with at least one of the following:

a. Symptoms and/or signs compatible with myocardial ischaemia
b. ECG changes compatible with myocardial ischaemia including new or presumed new ST-segment changes, T wave changes or left bundle branch block
c. The development of pathological Q waves on the ECG
d. Imaging evidence of new loss of viable myocardium
e. Identification of an intracoronary thrombus by angiography or postmortem [2]

WHAT IS TROPONIN?

Troponin is a subunit of the troponin–tropomyosin complex, part of the myofibrillar contractile apparatus. There are three forms of troponin: I, T and C. Troponin itself is not cardiac specific and is present within the contractile apparatus of both skeletal and cardiac muscle. The development of immunoassays for the cardiac isoform of troponins I and T has, however, yielded a highly cardiac-specific biomarker with very little skeletal muscle crossover.

There are many commercially available automated immunoassays for cardiac troponins I and T. An exhaustive list of currently available assays is available from the International Federation of Clinical Chemistry [3]. For diagnostic purposes, cardiac troponins I and T are essentially considered equivalent. There is some evidence that troponin I assays may yield fewer positive results outside of the context of AMI than troponin T [4]. However, the analytical characteristics of the cardiac troponin assay itself are far more important determinants of diagnostic accuracy than whether the assay targets troponin T or troponin I.

WHY IS THE DIAGNOSTIC CUT-OFF FOR AMI SET SO LOW?

Since 2000, international guidance has stipulated that AMI can be diagnosed when troponin levels rise above the 99th percentile of levels observed in apparently healthy individuals [1]. For many years, however, higher diagnostic cut-offs have been used in clinical practice. There were two reasons for setting the cut-off above the 99th percentile: firstly, a higher cut-off will yield higher diagnostic specificity and fewer 'false positive' results in patients who do not have AMI; and secondly, there were concerns about the precision of troponin assays at low levels. As troponin assays have improved, the issue of precision has largely been resolved. Some people have, however, remained concerned about the clinical significance of marginal troponin elevations.

There is now convincing evidence for the use of a cut-off set at the 99th percentile in apparently healthy individuals as recommended in international guidance. In an observational study, Body et al showed that minimal troponin rises above the 99th percentile upper reference limit independently and predicted major adverse cardiac events within 6 months [5].

More recently, Mills et al provided the first evidence that changing clinical protocols to diagnose AMI at lower cut-offs leads to improved outcomes for patients. They reported that an outdated troponin cut-off had been in clinical use to diagnose AMI at the Edinburgh Royal Infirmary (0.2 ng/mL, whereas the 99th percentile of the assay was 0.04 ng/mL). In an initial retrospective 'validation study' of 1038 patients, this group studied the prognosis of patients with minimal troponin elevations that were above the 99th percentile cut-off but below the diagnostic cut-off for AMI that was being used at that institution. They found that this group had a disproportionately high incidence of death or AMI at 1 year. The incidence was 39% among patients with troponin levels between 0.05 and 0.19 ng/mL, compared with 24% among patients whose troponin levels were ≥0.20 ng/mL [6].

Subsequently, they lowered the diagnostic cut-off that was used in practice such that patients with troponin levels above 0.05 ng/mL would be diagnosed with AMI and would receive the relevant treatment. After implementing this change, Mills' group re-evaluated clinical outcomes. They found that clinical outcomes remained unchanged for patients with troponin levels below the new diagnostic cut-off or above the previous cut-off. However, the patients with minimal troponin elevations – who had disproportionately bad outcomes in the validation phase and who were now being diagnosed with and treated for AMI – had significantly better outcomes such that the incidence of death or AMI had been reduced to 21% [6]. This provides the strongest evidence to date that accepting a lower diagnostic cut-off for cardiac troponin leads to better clinical outcomes for patients. Of course, it remains important to remember that the diagnosis of AMI requires not just a single troponin elevation but a rise and/or fall of cardiac troponin on serial sampling in conjunction with the appropriate clinical context.

HIGH-SENSITIVITY TROPONIN

Cardiac troponin has revolutionised the diagnosis of AMI, enabling detection of microscopic amounts of myocardial necrosis that had previously been impossible. However, the available tests are imperfect tools to enable its detection and quantification. Until recently, commercially available troponin assays have been subject to two important analytical limitations. Firstly, the precision of a biomarker assay determines the reliability of the results reported. With increasing precision, the results reported when re-testing the same sample for a number of times will be closer together. Precision is measured by the coefficient of variation (CV), which is equal to the mean value returned when testing a sample several times divided by its standard deviation. The CV tends to be higher (indicating lower precision) at lower troponin concentrations. For an assay to be acceptable according to contemporary international guidance, the CV should be <10% when the troponin concentration in the sample is equal to the 99th percentile in an apparently healthy population [2]. Historically, troponin assays have failed to achieve this standard.

Secondly, until recently it has not been possible to detect troponin levels in apparently healthy individuals. As such, the 99th percentile upper reference limit has been equal to the detection limit of the test. It has, therefore, been impossible to know whether detection of lesser troponin rises could lead to benefits for patients.

High-sensitivity troponin assays overcome both of these analytical limitations. In order for a troponin assay to be labelled as 'high sensitivity' it must, therefore, meet two criteria:
1. The CV must be <10% at the 99th percentile upper reference limit, i.e. the assays have improved precision
2. It must be possible to detect troponin levels in at least half of apparently healthy individuals, i.e. the assays have improved analytical sensitivity [7]

IMPORTANT TERMINOLOGY

In order to understand how high-sensitivity troponins can be optimally used in clinical practice, it is important to be aware of the definition of several important terms, discussed below [8]:

The limit of blank

This is essentially the highest level of troponin that we might reasonably expect to see reported if a sample containing no troponin is tested. It is calculated as the mean +1.645 standard deviations of the results obtained after repeated testing of a sample containing no troponin.

The limit of detection

This level is higher than the limit of blank (LoB). It is the lowest level of troponin that could be reliably distinguished from a sample containing no troponin. It is calculated as the mean +1.645 standard deviations of the results obtained after repeated testing of a sample containing a very low concentration of troponin.

The limit of quantification

This is defined at the lowest concentration at which certain precision criteria can be fulfilled. For a troponin assay, this is usually considered to be the lowest troponin concentration at which the CV is <10%.

Familiarity with these terms will be required in order to understand some of the novel clinical applications of high-sensitivity troponin assays, as described below.

CLINICAL IMPLICATIONS OF HIGH-SENSITIVITY TROPONIN ASSAYS

In addition to the analytical imperfections of commercially available assays, cardiac troponin has some important clinical limitations as a biomarker for the diagnosis of acute coronary syndromes that directly affect clinical care.

1. It takes several hours for troponin levels to rise in the bloodstream after the onset of myocardial injury. This necessitates serial sampling of a number of hours and means that the diagnosis of AMI cannot usually be 'ruled out' when patients first present to the hospital: a phenomenon known as 'troponin blindness'
2. Patients with unstable angina, who have symptomatic coronary plaque rupture or erosion, will have no detectable troponin rise even with serial sampling, which is a problem of 'troponin invisibility'

'Troponin blindness' and early 'rule out' strategies

The first of these issues (troponin blindness) means that many patients must be admitted to hospital for serial troponin testing before acute coronary syndromes can safely be 'ruled out'. This has substantial resource implications for health services. Chest pain is the most common reason for emergency hospital admission in England and Wales, accounting for over a quarter of acute medical admissions [9,10]. Of those who are initially suspected to have the diagnosis of an acute coronary syndrome, only a minority actually has that diagnosis. A strategy that could 'rule out' acute coronary syndromes without the requirement for serial sampling over a number of hours could enable patients to receive earlier reassurance about the nature of their symptoms, unburdening overcrowded emergency departments and substantially reducing resource utilisation for hospitals.

In 2009, the first reports of the diagnostic accuracy of high-sensitivity troponin tests when used to 'rule out' AMI at the time of first presentation to the hospital were published. In a landmark study of 786 patients with chest pain presenting to the emergency department, Reichlin et al showed that, using the high-sensitivity troponin T assay (Roche diagnostics), 95% of patients with AMI had positive results (above the 99th percentile upper reference limit) at the time of arrival in the emergency department. In comparison, only 83% of patients with AMI had a positive result using the previous generation of troponin T assay [11]. Such evidence shows how the use of high-sensitivity troponin assays will ameliorate the problem of 'troponin blindness' by reducing the proportion of patients with AMI whose troponin levels are normal at the time of presentation. However, because the strategy would miss 5% of AMIs this evidence also shows that serial sampling remains necessary before we can consider the diagnosis of AMI to be 'ruled out'.

However, with high-sensitivity troponin assays it may be possible to reduce the period of 'troponin blindness' by bringing forward the timing of serial samples. With the previous generations of troponin assay, it was necessary to undertake serial sampling 6–9 hours after arrival in the hospital or 12 hours after symptom onset before the diagnosis of AMI could be 'ruled out' [12,13]. The advent of high-sensitivity troponins has led to hope that AMI may be excluded by serial sampling within 2–3 hours of presentation.

In 2009, Keller et al evaluated a contemporary, sensitive assay (troponin I, Siemens Ultra, which has since failed to meet the criteria for being labelled as 'high sensitivity'). The sensitivity of this troponin I test when used at the time of arrival and 3 hours later was shown to be 100.0% [14]. A secondary analysis from the same study evaluating another troponin assay (Abbott ARCHITECT high-sensitivity troponin I), which does fulfil the criteria for being a 'high-sensitivity' assay, showed that testing 3 hours after admission and using the 99th percentile upper reference limit as a cut-off, the sensitivity was 98.2% [15]. This evidence led to a change in the wording of the universal definition of myocardial infarction in 2012, to state [2] the following.

'Blood samples should be for the measurement of cardiac troponin should be drawn on first assessment and repeated 3–6 hours later'.

The European Society of Cardiology and the National Institute for Health and Care Excellence in the United Kingdom have also recommended that an early rule out protocol incorporating testing on arrival and 3 hours later can be used when a high-sensitivity troponin assay is available [16,17].

Early rule out strategies using extremely low troponin cut-offs

The 3-hour rule out strategy will reduce the period of 'troponin blindness' but it still requires patients to stay in the hospital for at least 4 hours, allowing for the turnaround time of the tests. A strategy that would enable the diagnosis of AMI to be rapidly excluded using a single blood test would have great advantages. Using the conventional 99th percentile upper reference limit as a cut-off it is not possible to do this, even with a high-sensitivity assay. However, high-sensitivity troponin allows the detection of much smaller levels of troponin. If the cut-off was lowered such that patients with extremely low levels of troponin on arrival were considered to have AMI 'ruled out', we could avoid the need for serial sampling in a proportion of patients.

With the Roche high-sensitivity troponin T assay, setting the cut-off at the LoB of the assay (such that patients with completely undetectable levels of troponin would have AMI 'ruled out') has been shown to have 100% sensitivity for AMI using a single blood test at the time of arrival in the emergency department, regardless of the time from symptom onset [18]. By excluding AMI in patients with troponin levels below the LoB, further investigation could be avoided in a quarter of all patients. Using a slightly higher cut-off set at the limit of detection (5 ng/L), a Swedish group showed that 'ruling out' AMI in patients with an initial troponin level <5 ng/L and no evidence of ECG ischaemia would give a negative predictive value of 99.8% for AMI occurring within the next 30 days [19]. These strategies therefore have great promise as means of immediately excluding the diagnosis of AMI without the need for any serial sampling. However, there have been concerns about the precision of the assays at such low troponin concentrations [20]. To date, these concerns have precluded clinical implementation and mean that further evidence is likely to be required before these strategies are incorporated into international guidance.

Biomarkers as part of clinical decision rules

Clinical decision rules are tools designed to aid decision-making processes in clinical medicine. Usually, they are derived through original research using multivariate analysis. An advantage of clinical decision rules is that they can optimise the combination of biomarker levels with other clinical information, e.g. ECG findings or details of a patient's symptoms. There are several examples of clinical decision rules that could be used in patients presenting to the emergency department with symptoms that are compatible with an acute coronary syndrome.

The Thrombolysis in Myocardial Infarction (TIMI) risk score was originally derived to risk stratify patients who have a confirmed diagnosis of an acute coronary syndrome (see **Table 4.1**) [21]. It has since been shown to effectively risk stratify patients with suspected acute coronary syndromes in the emergency department [22]. Patients with a TIMI risk score of 0 who have normal troponin levels (below the 99th percentile upper reference limit) on arrival and 2 hours later could potentially have the diagnosis of acute coronary syndrome excluded. In the ADAPT trial, which included 1975 patients, this strategy could have enabled the early discharge of 20% of patients with suspected cardiac chest pain

Table 4.1 The Thrombolysis in Myocardial Infarction (TIMI) risk score*
Age >65 years
Current use of aspirin
At least three risk factors for coronary artery disease (hypertension, hyperlipidaemia, family history, tobacco smoking, diabetes mellitus)
Known coronary stenosis
Severe symptoms (at least two episodes in the preceding 24 hours)
ECG ischaemia
Troponin level >99th percentile
*1 point for each parameter. definitions may vary between studies.

with a sensitivity of 99.7% and a negative predictive value of 99.7% for major adverse cardiac events occurring within 30 days [23]. In a subsequent randomised controlled trial comparing the use of this strategy to routine care (including delayed troponin testing), the TIMI-based protocol allowed 19.3% of patients to be safely discharged within 6 hours, compared to 11.0% of patients who received standard care [24]. Having been subjected to a randomised controlled trial, therefore, this strategy could be used immediately in the clinical environment to facilitate early discharge, although the proportion of patients discharged early may be relatively modest.

The HEART score is an alternative clinical decision rule, which relies on information available at the time of arrival in the hospital (**Table 4.2**). This score was derived using the intuition of a cardiologist (Jacob Six) rather than through statistical analysis. However, its performance has been validated in several large cohort studies. In general, these studies support clinical use of the HEART score, reporting that the incidence of major adverse cardiac events within 30 days is below 2% for patients with a low HEART score (0–3 points) [25–27], although there have been reports that the HEART score has lower accuracy [28]. The results of an interventional trial that is currently recruiting will help to inform the field whether the HEART score is a safe and efficient tool to reduce unnecessary hospital admissions [29].

Another clinical decision rule that has recently been described is the Manchester Acute Coronary Syndromes (MACS) rule. This decision rule was derived by multivariate analysis in a cohort of 698 patients and subsequently validated in 463 patients at a separate centre [30]. The MACS rule incorporates eight variables including two biomarker levels (**Table 4.3**). The rule requires calibration for each troponin assay in order to optimise the diagnostic performance and considers each biomarker level to be a continuous variable.

Table 4.2 The HEART score*	
Category	**Score**
H: history	Highly suspicious: 2 points
	Moderately suspicious: 1 point
	Slightly or nonsuspicious: 0 point
E: ECG	Significant standard deviation: 2 points
	Nonspecific repolarisation abnormality: 1 point
	Normal: 0 point
A: age	≥65 years: 2 points
	46–64 years: 1 point
	≤45 years: 0 point
R: risk factors	≥3 risk factors or known atherosclerotic disease: 2 points
	1–2 risk factors: 1 point
	0 risk factor: 0 point
T: troponin	≥3 times upper reference limit: 2 points
	1–3 times upper reference limit: 1 point
	≤ upper reference limit: 0 point

*Patients with a score of 0–3 points are considered to be at 'low risk' and suitable for early discharge from the emergency department [29].

Thus, there is no single diagnostic cut-off but the MACS rule recognises that, with rising levels of each biomarker, there is a continuum of risk. Similar to the Global Registry of Acute Cardiac Events score, which is used to risk stratify patients with confirmed acute coronary syndromes, the MACS rule requires a computerised calculation. Patients are stratified into four risk groups based on this calculation. The 'very low risk' group includes 27% of all patients. In the validation study, none of these patients had an AMI and 1.6% developed a major adverse cardiac event within 30 days. As well as facilitating early discharge of patients from the emergency department and thus reduction of the need for unnecessary hospital admission, the MACS rule enables overall risk stratification. In the 'high risk' group (9.9% of all patients), over 95% of patients developed a major adverse cardiac event within 30 days. However, prior to widespread clinical implementation it will be important to gather further data on the likely impact of the rule when used in clinical practice, e.g. from interventional trials.

'Troponin invisibility' and unstable angina

With high-sensitivity troponin assays a greater proportion of patients will test positive for troponin. This appears to be particularly so for the high-sensitivity troponin T assay (manufactured by Roche). With the previous generation of troponin T assay, the 99th percentile upper reference limit was 0.01 ng/mL or 10 ng/L. If a sample had been shown to contain 10 ng/L of troponin using that assay and was re-tested using the newer, high-sensitivity assay, the equivalent result using the new assay is likely to be approximately 35 ng/L. This means that the apparent troponin concentration is higher using the high-sensitivity assay [31]. As the 99th percentile upper reference limit for the high-sensitivity assay is 14 ng/L, those patients who have troponin levels between 14 and 35 ng/L using the high-sensitivity assay will now test positive, whereas they would previously have had negative (or normal) troponin levels. In patients with acute coronary syndromes, this leads to a greater proportion of patients being diagnosed with non-ST elevation myocardial infarction (NSTEMI), whereas they would previously have been diagnosed with unstable angina [32]. As such, the apparent incidence of NSTEMI will increase and that of unstable angina will decrease. This has led some people to believe that unstable angina will cease to exist as a diagnosis as troponin assays become increasingly sensitive in the future.

Table 4.3 The Manchester Acute Coronary Syndromes (MACS) decision rule for suspected cardiac chest pain*
High-sensitivity troponin T
Heart-type fatty acid binding protein
ECG ischaemia
Pain in association with vomiting
Sweating observed in the emergency department
Hypotension on arrival (systolic blood pressure <100 mmHg)
Worsening angina

*Each variable is entered into a computer. High-sensitivity troponin T is entered in ng/L; heart-type fatty acid binding protein in ng/mL. Categorical variables are considered to be either present (1) or absent (0). The computer then calculates an estimated probability that the patient will develop a major adverse cardiac event within 30 days. Based on this, patients are stratified into four risk groups. The 'very low' risk group can be immediately discharged from hospital.

Causes of troponin elevation

At the same time, as patients with acute coronary syndromes are more likely to test positive for troponin, when a high-sensitivity assay is used, it is equally true that more patients who do not have an acute coronary syndrome will test positive. It is tempting to label such results as 'false positives' but it is important to remember that troponin is a marker of myocardial injury rather than specifically being a marker of AMI. As such, any cause of myocardial injury will lead to a troponin elevation. Some of these alternative causes of troponin elevation are listed in **Table 4.4**.

On encountering a patient with a troponin elevation, the first priority is to attempt to distinguish those patients who have AMI from those who have another cause for their troponin elevation. In this regard, the clinical context is the most important consideration. Firstly, we need to understand whether the patient is likely to have a chronic troponin elevation. A number of factors are known to influence a patient's baseline troponin level. Advancing age, male gender, renal dysfunction, left ventricular dysfunction and underlying cardiovascular disease are all known to cause chronic troponin elevations. These patients have a worse long-term prognosis but the troponin rise is not caused by an AMI. In a reference ranging study, it has been shown that the 99th percentile upper reference limit for the high-sensitivity troponin T assay is 14 ng/L (as published by the manufacturer) only if the reference population excludes patients with evidence left ventricular dysfunction, cardiovascular disease and renal disease. In the undifferentiated population, the 99th percentile was found to be 29.9 ng/L [33]. This is useful to clinicians as it informs us about the magnitude of troponin elevation we might expect at baseline in patients who have comorbidities such as left ventricular dysfunction. In patients with chronic kidney disease, troponin levels may be even higher at baseline. The 95th percentile in apparently healthy patients with chronic kidney disease from stages 3 to 5 has been shown to be as high as 139 ng/L [34].

Assessing a rise and/or fall of troponin

In a patient who has an elevated troponin level, we must also determine whether the level changes over time. In order to diagnose AMI we must demonstrate that a patient has a rise and/or fall of cardiac troponin [2]. A patient with a troponin elevation that does not change over time is likely to have a chronic troponin elevation but not AMI. This means that serial sampling is necessary to determine the change or 'δ' troponin over time. International guidance now recommends that samples should be drawn 3–6 hours apart but do not precisely define a 'rise and/or fall' of cardiac troponin [2].

Table 4.4 Causes of troponin elevation	
Type 1 myocardial infarction	Type 2 myocardial infarction
Heart failure	Renal failure
Pulmonary embolism	Critical illness
Myocarditis	Aortic dissection
Hypertrophic obstructive cardiomyopathy	Cardiac contusion
Arrhythmias	Subarachnoid haemorrhage
Takotsubo cardiomyopathy	Extreme exertion
Burns	Normal biological variation

The National Academy of Clinical Biochemistry originally proposed that a 20% change in troponin levels on serial sampling is necessary to make the diagnosis of AMI [35]. However, as there is such heterogeneity between troponin assays, the appropriate δ should be defined for each individual assay. There is evidence that the 20% δ may not be optimal for diagnosis. For example, Mueller et al demonstrated that only 75.2% of patients with NSTEMI will develop a δ >20%, whereas 62.4% of patients who do not have a diagnosis of an acute coronary syndrome will develop a δ of >20% on serial sampling [36]. One of the key limitations of this approach is that the 20% criteria are a 'relative' δ. This means that patients who have a troponin level just above the 99th percentile can develop a 20% δ on serial sampling despite there being only a small absolute change. Conversely, a patient with an extremely high troponin level may not develop a 20% δ despite a very large absolute change on serial sampling, e.g. a patient with a troponin level of 10 ng/L at baseline and 15 ng/L at 6 hours would be diagnosed with AMI using a relative δ (50%), despite having a very small absolute change in troponin (5 ng/L) that could be caused by the imprecision of the assay. A second patient, however, does not meet the 20% criterion despite having an extremely high troponin level (2000 ng/L at baseline; 2200 ng/L at 6 hours) and an absolute change of 200 ng/L on serial sampling (relative δ: 10%).

Thus, using an 'absolute' δ (the absolute difference in troponin levels on serial sampling) may have some advantages. This approach has shown to have higher diagnostic accuracy for AMI than the use of relative ds. For the high-sensitivity troponin T assay, the optimal δ was shown to be an absolute change of ≥9.2 ng/L [36].

Type 2 myocardial infarction

When a patient is shown to have a rise and/or fall of cardiac troponin it is important to again consider the clinical context. We need to differentiate those patients whose AMI has been caused by a primary plaque rupture, erosion or dissection (type 1 AMI) from those in whom a condition other than coronary artery disease has caused an imbalance between myocardial oxygen supply and demand (e.g. AMI caused by severe anaemia, critical illness or haemorrhage). The latter may, e.g. be caused by arrhythmias, critical illness or by coronary artery spasm. Patients with type 2 AMI have a disproportionately high mortality rate [37] but may not benefit from the same antiplatelet and antithrombotic treatment as has been shown to benefit patients with type 1 AMI. Treatment of the underlying condition is likely to have greater importance, particularly in the acute phase.

ALTERNATIVE BIOMARKERS

CK-MB and myoglobin

CK-MB and myoglobin have been proposed as 'early markers' of myocardial injury that could identify patients who present early after symptom onset, during the period of 'troponin blindness'. However, these biomarkers lack specificity. Compared to the use of a contemporary troponin assay alone, they do not increase sensitivity for AMI but they reduce specificity. This means that hospital admission can be avoided for fewer patients [23,38]. In a multi-centre randomised controlled trial, the use of a multimarker panel (CK-MB, myoglobin and troponin) on arrival and 90 minutes later was compared to standard care. In this trial, the proportion of patients that was safely discharged from hospital increased [39]. However, driven by an increase in coronary care utilisation, healthcare resource use also increased (perhaps as a function of the lack of specificity of CK-MB and myoglobin) meaning that the strategy was not cost-effective [40].

Heart-type fatty acid binding protein (H-FABP)

This is a cytosolic protein that facilitates intracellular fatty acid transport and is abundantly expressed within cardiac myocytes. Being a cytosolic protein with relatively low molecular weight, theoretically, we would expect H-FABP to be released into the bloodstream early after the onset of myocardial injury. Indeed, the sensitivity of H-FABP has been shown to be superior to the sensitivity of cardiac troponin (using a standard, nonhigh-sensitivity assay) when measured within 4 hours after symptom onset [41]. However, a meta-analysis of 16 studies (including 3709 patients) demonstrated that the sensitivity of H-FABP, when used alone, is insufficient (84%) to rule out AMI when used alone [42]. The sensitivity can be improved when combined with troponin but, again, a single test would be insufficient to rule out AMI unless used selectively in a low-risk population [43]. When used in combination with a high-sensitivity troponin assay, performance may improve still further. In a study of 1818 patients an area under the receiver operating characteristic curve of 0.97 has been reported for this combination. However, the best current evidence for clinical use is when H-FABP is used as part of the MACS decision rule, which combines H-FABP with high-sensitivity troponin and six other variables that were found to independently predict major adverse cardiac events within 30 days.

Copeptin

Copeptin is the C-terminal part of the precursor peptide for arginine vasopressin (AVP; also known as antidiuretic hormone) and is used as a surrogate marker for AVP. It is released early after the onset of AMI in response to haemodynamic stimuli. The combination of AVP and troponin has attracted significant attention in the medial literature as another strategy that could facilitate the early 'rule out' of AMI in the emergency department. A systematic review of 14 studies including 9244 patients showed that, in combination with troponin, copeptin has a sensitivity of 90.5%, a specificity of 68.6% and a negative predictive value of 97.0% [44]. This may be considered insufficient to safely exclude a diagnosis as important as AMI. However, in a recent randomised controlled trial, 902 patients were randomised to receive standard care or care guided by an accelerated discharge protocol that would enable discharge if the troponin and copeptin levels were normal on arrival. In that trial, the rates of major adverse cardiac events were similar in each group. Of the patients who had normal troponin and copeptin levels who were discharged from hospital, the incidence of major adverse cardiac events was low (0.6%) [45].

SUMMARY AND FUTURE DIRECTIONS

Cardiac troponin has revolutionised the diagnosis of AMI and enables the detection of infarction that was not previously possible. Over time, cardiac troponin assays have improved both in terms of analytical sensitivity (detection of lower concentrations) and precision (reliability of the results). This has enabled us to diagnose AMI much sooner and to identify more patients who have unstable coronary disease, thus reducing the problems of 'troponin invisibility' and 'troponin blindness'. By using innovative strategies such as clinical decision rules, novel low troponin cut-offs or emerging alternative biomarkers such as copeptin or H-FABP, it may be possible to reduce these problems still further. In order to 'rule in' AMI using biomarkers, current international guidance mandates serial sampling to a rise and/or fall in cardiac troponin levels. Recent evidence strongly suggests that an absolute change in troponin is superior to a relative change in troponin on serial sampling for AMI diagnosis but the precise change needs to be defined for each individual assay. Finally, while cardiac biomarkers are improving, they cannot remove the need for a clinician. As there are many alternative causes of troponin elevations, cardiac troponin alone can never be used to diagnose AMI. Taking account of the clinical context in order to anticipate the patient's baseline level of troponin and to seek possible explanations for an acute troponin rise other than AMI is essential.

Future work will need to focus on validating the 'rapid rule out' strategies outlined above, defining the optimum δ troponin for each assay in clinical use and developing novel algorithms that may be used to supplement clinical judgement in differentiating patients with troponin elevations caused by AMI from those that are not caused by AMI.

Key points for clinical practice

- A change in cardiac troponin level is central to the diagnosis of AMI.
- High-sensitivity troponin detects smaller AMIs than was previously possible. Some patients who were previously diagnosed with unstable angina will now be diagnosed with NSTEMI.
- With high-sensitivity troponin, two tests taken 3 hours apart can be used to 'rule out' AMI.
- Risk scores that take account of other clinical information (e.g. the HEART score, MACS rule or ADAPT protocol) could enable AMI to be 'ruled out' sooner.
- The detection of a rise and/or fall of troponin on serial sampling is necessary to 'rule in' AMI. Absolute changes in troponin are superior to relative changes but the required change on serial sampling must be defined for each troponin assay.
- There are many causes of troponin elevation other than AMI. Taking account of the clinical context is crucial.
- In a patient with a raised troponin level, it is also important to differentiate between type 1 and type 2 AMI.
- There is growing evidence that alternative biomarkers such as copeptin or H-FABP may enhance risk stratification when used in combination with troponin.

REFERENCES

1. The Joint European Society of Cardiology/American College of Cardiology Committee. Myocardial infarction redefined – a consensus document of The Joint European Society of Cardiology/American College of Cardiology Committee for the redefinition of myocardial infarction. Eur Heart J 2000; 21:1502–1513.
2. Thygesen K, Alpert JS, Jaffe AS, et al. Third universal definition of myocardial infarction. J Am Coll Cardiol 2012; 60:1581–1598.
3. International Federation of Clinical Chemistry and Laboratory Medicine. Troponin assay analytical characteristics. Italy: IFCC, 2013. http://www.ifcc.org/ifcc-scientific-division/documents-of-the-sd/troponinassayanalyticalcharacteristics2013/. (Last accessed 22 December 2014.)
4. Cullen L, Aldous S, Than M, et al. Comparison of high sensitivity troponin T and I assays in the diagnosis of non-ST elevation acute myocardial infarction in emergency patients with chest pain. Clin Biochem 2014; 47:321–326.

5. Body R, Carley S, McDowell G, Ferguson J, Mackway-Jones K. Diagnosing acute myocardial infarction with troponins: how low can you go? Emerg Med J 2009; 27:292–296.
6. Mills NL, Churchhouse AMD, Lee KK, et al. Implementation of a sensitive troponin I assay and risk of recurrent myocardial infarction and death in patients with suspected acute coronary syndrome. JAMA 2011; 305:1210–1216.
7. Apple FS, Collinson PO, The IFCC Task Force on Clinical Applications of Cardiac Biomarkers. Analytical characteristics of high-sensitivity cardiac troponin assays. Clin Chem 2011; 58:54–61.
8. Armbruster D, Pry T. Limit of blank, limit of detection and limit of quantitation. Clin Biochem Rev 2008; 29:S49–S52.
9. The Health and Social Care Information Centre. Primary diagnosis, 3 characters table. Hospital Episode Statistics, Admitted Patient Care – England, 2012–13. Leeds, UK. HSCIC, 2013. http://www.hesonline.nhs.uk. (Last accessed 25 November 2013.)
10. Goodacre S, Cross E, Arnold J, et al. The health care burden of acute chest pain. Heart 2005; 91:229–230.
11. Reichlin T, Hochholzer W, Bassetti S, et al. Early diagnosis of myocardial infarction with sensitive cardiac troponin assays. N Engl J Med 2009; 361:858–867.
12. Thygesen K, Alpert JS, White HD (on behalf of the Joint ESC/ACCF/AHA/WHF Task Force for the Redefinition of Myocardial Infarction). Universal definition of myocardial infarction. Circulation 2007; 116:2634–2653.
13. National Clinical Guideline Centre for Acute and Chronic Conditions. Chest Pain of Recent Onset: Assessment and Diagnosis of Recent Onset Chest Pain or Discomfort of Suspected Cardiac Origin. NICE Guideline. London: NICE, 2010.
14. Keller T, Zeller T, Peetz D, et al. Sensitive troponin I assay in early diagnosis of acute myocardial infarction. N Engl J Med 2009; 361:868–877.
15. Keller T, Zeller T, Ojeda F, et al. Serial changes in highly sensitive troponin I assay and early diagnosis of myocardial infarction. JAMA 2011; 306:2684–2693.
16. Hamm CW, Bassand J-P, Agewall S (Authors/Task Force Members)et al. ESC Guidelines for the management of acute coronary syndromes in patients presenting without persistent ST-segment elevation: The Task Force for the management of acute coronary syndromes (ACS) in patients presenting without persistent ST-segment elevation of the European Society of Cardiology (ESC). Eur Heart J 2011; 32:2999–3054.
17. National Institute for Health and Care Excellence. Myocardial infarction (acute) – early rule out using high sensitivity troponin tests (Elecsys Troponin T high-sensitive, ARCHITECT STAT High Sensitive Troponin-I and Accu-TnI+3 assays). Report No.: NICE in development [GID-DT18]. London: Nice, 2014. https://www.nice. org.uk/Guidance/InDevelopment/GID-DT18/Documents. (Last accessed 30 July 2014.)
18. Body R, Carley S, McDowell G, et al. Rapid exclusion of acute myocardial infarction in patients with undetectable troponin using a high-sensitivity assay. J Am Coll Cardiol 2011; 58:1332–1329.
19. Bandstein N, Ljung R, Johansson M, Holzmann MJ. Undetectable high sensitivity troponin T level in the emergency department and risk of myocardial infarction. J Am Coll Cardiol 2014; 63:2569–2678.
20. Kavsak P, Worster A. Dichotomizing high sensitivity cardiac troponin T results and important analytical considerations. J Am Coll Cardiol 2012; 59:1570.
21. Antman EM, Cohen M, Bernink PJLM, et al. The TIMI risk score for unstable angina/non-ST elevation MI: A method for prognostication and therapeutic decision making. JAMA 2000; 284:835–842.
22. Hess EP, Agarwal D, Chandra S, et al. Diagnostic accuracy of the TIMI risk score in patients with chest pain in the emergency department: a meta-analysis. Can Med Assoc J 2010; 182:1039–1044.
23. Than M, Cullen L, Aldous S, et al. 2-Hour accelerated diagnostic protocol to assess patients with chest pain symptoms using contemporary troponins as the only biomarker: the ADAPT trial. J Am Coll Cardiol 2012; 59:2091–2098.
24. Than M, Aldous S, Lord SJ, et al. A 2-hour diagnostic protocol for possible cardiac chest pain in the emergency department: a randomized clinical trial. JAMA Intern Med 2014; 174:51–58.
25. Six AJ, Cullen L, Backus BE, et al. The HEART score for the assessment of patients with chest pain in the emergency department: a multinational validation study. Crit Pathw Cardiol 2013; 12:121–126.
26. Backus BE, Six AJ, Kelder JC, et al. A prospective validation of the HEART score for chest pain patients at the emergency department. Int J Cardiol 2013; 168:2153–2158.
27. Backus, BE, Six, AJ, Kelder, JC, et al. Chest pain in the Emergency Room: a multicentre validation of the HEART score. Crit Pathw Cardiol 2010; 9:164–169.
28. Mahler SA, Hiestand BC, Goff DC, Hoekstra JW, Miller CD. Can the HEART score safely reduce stress testing and cardiac imaging in patients at low risk for major adverse cardiac events? Crit Pathw Cardiol 2011; 10:128–133.

29. Poldervaart JM, Reitsma JB, Koffijberg H, et al. The impact of the HEART risk score in the early assessment of patients with acute chest pain: design of a stepped wedge, cluster randomised trial. BMC Cardiovasc Disord 2013; 13:77.

30. Body R, Carley S, McDowell G, et al. The Manchester Acute Coronary Syndromes (MACS) decision rule for suspected cardiac chest pain: derivation and external validation. Heart 2014; 100:1462–1468.

31. Giannitsis E, Kurz K, Hallermayer K, et al. Analytical validation of a high-sensitivity cardiac troponin T assay. Clin Chem 2010; 56:254–261.

32. Giannitsis E, Becker M, Kurz K, et al. High-sensitivity cardiac troponin T for early prediction of evolving non-ST-segment elevation myocardial infarction in patients with suspected acute coronary syndrome and negative troponin results on admission. Clin Chem 2010; 56:642–650.

33. Collinson PO, Heung YM, Gaze D, et al. Influence of population selection on the 99th percentile reference value for cardiac troponin assays. Clin Chem 2012; 58:219–225.

34. Chotivanawan T, Krittayaphong R. Normal range of serum highly-sensitive troponin-T in patients with chronic kidney disease stage 3-5. J Med Assoc Thai 2012; 95:S127–S132.

35. NACB Writing Group, Wu AHB, Jaffe AS, et al. National Academy of Clinical Biochemistry laboratory medicine practice guidelines: use of cardiac troponin and B-type natriuretic peptide or N-terminal proB-type natriuretic peptide for etiologies other than acute coronary syndromes and heart failure. Clin Chem 2007; 53:2086–2096.

36. Mueller M, Biener M, Vafaie M, et al. Absolute and relative kinetic changes of high-sensitivity cardiac troponin T in acute coronary syndrome and in patients with increased troponin in the absence of acute coronary syndrome. Clin Chem 2011; 58:209–218.

37. Saaby L, Poulsen TS, Diederichsen ACP, et al. Mortality rate in type 2 myocardial infarction: observations from an unselected hospital cohort. Am J Med 2014; 127:295–302.

38. Than M, Cullen L, Reid CM, et al. A 2-h diagnostic protocol to assess patients with chest pain symptoms in the Asia-Pacific region (ASPECT): a prospective observational validation study. Lancet 2011; 377:1077–1084.

39. Goodacre S, Cross L, Lewis C (on behalf of the ESCAPE Research Team). The ESCAPE trial: Effectiveness and safety of chest pain assessment to prevent emergency admissions. Emerg Med J 2007; 24:A5.

40. Fitzgerald P, Goodacre SW, Cross E, Dixon S. Cost-effectiveness of point-of-care biomarker assessment for suspected myocardial infarction: the randomized assessment of treatment using panel assay of cardiac markers (RATPAC) trial. Acad Emerg Med 2011; 18:488–495.

41. McCann CJ, Glover BM, Menown IBA, et al. Novel biomarkers in early diagnosis of acute myocardial infarction compared with cardiac troponin T. Eur Heart J 2008; 29:2843–2850.

42. Bruins Slot MHE, Reitsma JB, Rutten FH, Hoes AW, van der Heijden GJMG. Heart-type fatty acid-binding protein in the early diagnosis of acute myocardial infarction: a systematic review and meta-analysis. Heart 2010; 96:1957–1963.

43. Body R, McDowell G, Carley S, et al. A FABP-ulous "rule out" strategy? Heart fatty acid binding protein and troponin for rapid exclusion of acute myocardial infarction. Resuscitation 2011; 82:1041–1046.

44. Lipinski MJ, Escárcega RO, D'Ascenzo F, et al. A systematic review and collaborative meta-analysis to determine the incremental value of copeptin for rapid rule-out of acute myocardial infarction. Am J Cardiol 2014; 113:1581–1591.

45. Mockel M, Searle J, Hamm C, et al. Early discharge using single cardiac troponin and copeptin testing in patients with suspected acute coronary syndrome (ACS): a randomized, controlled clinical process study. Eur Heart J. 2015; 36:369–376. http://eurheartj.oxfordjournals.org/cgi/doi/10.1093/eurheartj/ehu178. (Last accessed 17 June 2014.)

Chapter 5

HIV and coronary heart disease

Mosepele Mosepele, Virginia A Triant

INTRODUCTION

Coronary heart disease (CHD) is increasingly recognised as an important complication in chronic HIV infection. HIV is associated with an estimated 1.5–2-fold increased risk of CHD. Both traditional cardiovascular (CVD) and novel HIV-related risk factors contribute to this excess CVD risk among HIV-infected patients. While traditional CVD risk factors are increased among HIV-infected patients, they do not fully account for the increased risk observed. Chronic inflammation and immune activation are increasingly recognised as key factors contributing to CHD risk in HIV. Understanding of the role of antiretroviral therapy (ART) in CHD risk has evolved, with current data suggesting that treating HIV reduces CHD risk and that the benefit of the concomitant reduction in inflammation outweighs possible proatherogenic effects of individual medications. While treating traditional CHD risk factors is generally recommended, HIV-infected patients are less likely to receive guideline-concordant care with respect to CHD risk reduction compared with non-HIV-infected patients. Guidelines designed for the general population, however, are not always applicable in the setting of HIV and should be understood within the broader context of HIV-specific risk factors for CHD which are not reflected in the guidelines.

EPIDEMIOLOGY OF HIV-ASSOCIATED CHD

Multiple longitudinal cohorts in North America and Europe over the past decade have reported (**Table 5.1**) that HIV infection confers an overall 1.5–2-fold or higher risk of CHD compared with appropriate non-HIV control groups [1–8]. This increased risk has been shown to persist despite accounting for traditional CVD risk factors and ART. CHD risk has also been shown to be increased with lower CD4 cell count or higher HIV RNA [7]. The relative risk (RR) of CHD (comparing HIV with non-HIV individuals) is higher in women and in younger age groups [3], suggesting that the effect of HIV is more pronounced in patients typically considered to have low CHD risk. The medium-to-long-term risks of CVD in large HIV populations in resource-limited settings, such as sub-Saharan Africa, remain unknown. Although there is a lack of similar cohorts in resource-limited settings, there is justifiable concern that CHD will pose a significant health burden to this population, particularly to those with lower nadir CD4 counts in the setting of different national ART guideline treatment thresholds or limited access to antiretroviral drugs [9].

Mosepele Mosepele MD, Harvard T.H. Chan School of Public Health, University of Boston, Boston, USA

Virginia A Triant MD MPH, Division of Infectious Diseases and General Medicine, Massachusetts General Hospital, Boston, USA.
Email: vtriant@mgh.harvard.edu (for correspondence)

Table 5.1 Studies reporting associations between HIV and coronary heart disease

Study	Year	Population	N (HIV)	Primary result	Effect size
Klein	2002	Kaiser	4159	MI and CHD in HIV vs. control	1.5 (MI) 1.7 (CHD)
Currier	2003	CA Medicaid	28513	CHD in HIV (age 18–33) vs. control	2.06
Triant	2007	Partners	3851	MI in HIV vs. control	1.75
Obel	2007	Danish cohort	3953	CHD in HIV (on ART) vs. control	2.12
Lang	2010	FHDH	74958	MI in HIV vs. 3 population registries	1.5
Durand	2011	Quebec	7053	MI in HIV vs. 4:1 matched control	2.11
Freiberg	2013	VA	27350	MI in HIV vs. 2:1 matched control	1.48
Silverberg	2014	Kaiser	22081	MI and CHD in HIV vs. 10:1 matched control	1.4

ART, antiretroviral therapy; CHD, coronary heart disease; MI, myocardial infarction.

HIV-infected women and CHD

In contrast to the general population, HIV-infected women appear to have a relatively higher risk of CHD compared with men. Acute myocardial infarction (AMI) RR was 3 versus 1.4 for women median age 36 versus men median age 38 years in a health-care system-based study [3], and sex- and age-standardised morbidity ratio of AMI was 2.7 (95% CI 1.8–3.9) for women versus 1.4 (95% CI 1.3–1.6) for men in a large French cohort [5]. This heightened risk among women is concerning because women – particularly younger women – are typically considered to be low risk for CHD. Moreover, women make up almost two thirds of the HIV-infected patient population in sub-Saharan Africa, the epicentre of the HIV epidemic.

HIV–hepatitis co-infection and CHD

HIV-infected patients who are co-infected with hepatitis C virus are generally considered to be at a higher risk for CHD compared with HIV-monoinfected patients in most, but not all, studies examining the association [10]. However, HIV and hepatitis B virus co-infection, which is more prevalent in resource-limited settings, has not been shown to confer an increased risk of CHD in European cohorts.

HIV and CHD in resource-limited settings

There are no studies that have specifically explored the association between HIV and CHD in resource-limited settings [11]. However, multiple studies have reported high prevalence of risk factors for CHD among adults and adolescents infected with HIV, raising the possibility that CHD may also be common in this patient population [9]. Some studies have suggested an association between HIV and stroke in the sub-Saharan African setting [12]. With over 90% of the global HIV-infected patient population concentrated in sub-Saharan Africa, research into the association between HIV and CHD in this population is urgently required.

PATHOPHYSIOLOGY OF HIV-ASSOCIATED CHD

HIV-associated CHD is a multifactorial process driven both by traditional CHD risk factors and by novel factors related to HIV and its associated chronic inflammation.

Traditional risk factors for CHD

Traditional CHD risk factors including insulin resistance/diabetes, smoking, atherogenic dyslipidaemia and hypertension are common among HIV-infected patients across different geographical settings [13]; however, they remain poorly recognised and managed [14]. Smoking is extremely prevalent among HIV-infected patients, with a recent study demonstrating that HIV-infected patients lose more life years to smoking than to HIV. Dyslipidaemia is common, and HIV populations are characterised by low value of high-density lipoprotein (HDL) and elevated triglycerides. As in HIV-negative controls, a family history of CHD contributes to increased risk of CHD among HIV-infected patients. The implication of these findings is that failure to address traditional risk factors for CHD among HIV-infected patients will contribute to excess CHD morbidity in this patient population.

HIV replication and inflammation

HIV replication and inflammation were initially linked to increased risk of CHD in the landmark Strategies in the Management of ART (SMART) trial, a trial evaluating continuous versus intermittent ART, the primary outcome being recurrent opportunistic infection or death [15]. Contrary to expectation, in secondary analyses, participants in the ART treatment interruption arm (intermittent HIV replication) were more likely to experience CVD events compared with those on uninterrupted ART (continuous HIV suppression; hazard ratio = 1.6, CI 1.0–2.5, $P = 0.05$) [16]. Moreover, the inflammatory markers, interleukin 6 (IL-6) and d-dimer, increased 1 month after treatment interruption and baseline high-sensitivity C-reactive protein, IL-6 and d-dimer were strongly correlated to overall mortality [17]. This observation of excess CHD risk in relation to active HIV replication could, in part, be explained by evidence of decreased vascular dysfunction following initiation of ART. Although CHD was not the primary end point and the number of CHD events was small, the finding was significant in that it was the first to suggest that CHD risk from ongoing viral replication and associated inflammation outweighs potential proatherogenic effects of individual ART medications.

Immune dysregulation

HIV infection has deleterious effects on the immune system, and increased risk of CHD has been linked both to clinically measured CD4 T cell depletion and to other forms of immune dysregulation, such as T-cell activation and senescence. Both T-cell activation and senescence have been hypothesised to be in part driven by chronic gastrointestinal microbial translocation and cytomegalovirus co-infection [18].

Among HIV-infected patients, CD4 nadir below 200 cells per microlitre is an independent risk factor for CHD [19,20]. However, there does not seem to be excess CHD risk among HIV-infected patients with CD4 T cell nadir ≥ 500 cell per microlitre when compared with HIV-uninfected controls (after adjusting for traditional risk factors for CHD) [8]. These results from the Kaiser Permanente cohort study from 13 years of follow-up represent the most recent strong evidence for initiating ART at CD4 T cell count over 500 cells per microlitre for CHD risk reduction.

The role of T-cell activation, as measured by CD38+HLA-DR+ CD4+ T cells, in HIV infection remains unresolved, with some studies showing no evidence of association with subclinical CVD and some showing some evidence of association with subclinical CVD such as carotid intima thickness or arterial stiffness. None has shown a direct link to occurrence of CHD, although such studies are difficult to perform owing to the large number of patients and the long clinical follow-up required. Some possible contributors to T-cell activation among HIV-infected patients include cytomegalovirus and varicella zoster virus co-infection as well as chronic gastrointestinal microbial translocation. More recently, monocyte activation has emerged as a potential mechanistic pathway in HIV-associated CVD. A monocyte activation marker, soluble CD163, has been linked to high-risk coronary atherosclerosis plaque and arterial inflammation [21]. Like T-cell activation, T-cell senescence, as measured by CD28– and/or CD57+ cells and possibly considered a marker of accelerated ageing in HIV, has been associated with subclinical CVD such as carotid artery stiffness. Taken together, these findings indicate that immune dysfunction contributes to the establishment or progression of subclinical CVD in HIV.

High-risk atherosclerotic plaque features and arterial inflammation

HIV infection is associated with prevalent and severe asymptomatic coronary atherosclerosis [22]. When compared with age and traditional CVD-risk-matched HIV-negative controls, HIV-infected patients are significantly more likely to have features of vulnerable coronary atherosclerotic plaque: more prevalent low attenuation, spotty calcification and positive remodelling [23]. In the general population, these plaque features are associated with acute coronary syndrome (ACS) even among asymptomatic patients.

Arterial inflammation is considered the primary pathologic process in the development of atherosclerosis and subsequently of CHD. In a study of HIV-infected patients with atherosclerosis demonstrated on coronary angiography in whom arterial inflammation was investigated using 18flourine-2-deoxy-D-glucose positron emission tomography (PET), arterial inflammation based on the finding of high aortic target–background ratio was increased in HIV-infected participants and associated with markers of monocyte activation [24].

Endothelial reactivity and arterial stiffness

Endothelial dysfunction is associated with development of atherosclerosis and subsequent CVD events (including nonfatal ACS) in the general population. HIV infection has also been associated with reduced endothelial reactivity. This association is strongest among HIV-infected patients with known cardiac disease such as myocardial infarction. In some HIV cohorts, HIV-associated endothelial dysfunction improves following ART initiation, even though this dysfunction may initially be more strongly associated with traditional

CVD risk factors than HIV-specific factors (CD4 count, viral replication) among ART-naïve patients [25]. Modification of HIV-associated endothelial dysfunction with ACS agents such as ranolazine or nitrates has not been directly studied. CD4 nadir <200 has also been associated with increased arterial stiffness, while initiating ART at CD4 counts >200 is associated with decreased arterial stiffness [26].

Platelet activity and prothrombotic state

Because platelet activation and aggregation is a key step in the formation of occlusive thrombus following plaque rupture, platelet activity has been studied among HIV-infected patients. In vivo studies revealed that HIV-infected patients have increased platelet activity compared with HIV-uninfected controls. While increased platelet activity has not been linked directly to development of ACS among HIV-infected patients, abacavir exposure results in transient increase in platelet activating factor levels, while tenofovir-containing ART does not [27]. This observation has led to the hypothesis that increased platelet activity may contribute to possible increased risk of ACS among HIV-infected patients on abacavir-containing ART that has been observed in some HIV observational cohorts. A recent small experimental study concluded that 1-week exposure to low-dose aspirin can result in a decrease in both platelet activation and immune activation among HIV-infected patients [28]. Larger prospective studies are needed to establish the degree of clinical benefit of aspirin as primary prophylaxis for CHD among HIV-infected patients.

Antiretroviral therapy

Current consensus suggests that the overall benefit of ART exceeds the potential risk of CHD from individual potentially proatherogenic medications, such that all HIV-infected patients should be initiated on ART irrespective of CD4 count [29].

Increased risk of CHD has been described for first-generation protease inhibitors (PIs) such as indinavir and lopinavir/ritonavir [30], and for the nucleoside reverse transcriptase inhibitor (NRTI) abacavir [31] in the Data collection on Adverse events of anti-HIV Drugs (D:A:D) study. Secondary analysis of randomised trial data (not designed to assess CVD risk due to ART) did not find an increased risk of CHD from first-generation PI exposure, and meta-analyses have not confirmed the association [32]. For all practical purposes, these data are largely historical, as indinavir and nelfinavir are rarely used in clinical practice while use of lopinavir/ritonavir in resource-limited settings will probably be reduced significantly when second-generation PIs (e.g. atazanavir and darunavir) and non-NRTIs (e.g. rilpivirine) become widely available. Second-generation PIs such as atazanavir have not been associated with increased risk for CHD after 3 years of follow-up [33], suggesting that the PI/CHD risk association is not a PI-class wide effect, but rather, is probably limited to older PIs (**Table 5.2**).

In contrast, the association between abacavir and CHD risk remains controversial. Some observational data and secondary analyses of randomised controlled trial (RCT) data confirmed the D:A:D finding of an increased risk of CHD following abacavir exposure while others, including a US Food and Drug Administration meta-analysis, have not confirmed the association [32,34]. In an attempt to identify pathophysiologic clues to understand better the conflicting data on abacavir and CVD, multiple studies have investigated possible mechanisms or causal pathways (endothelial dysfunction, arterial stiffness, inflammation and platelet activation) and have shown mixed results, failing to resolve this controversy.

ART class	ART agent	Preferred	Avoid
Table 5.2 Preferred antiretroviral therapy agents to minimise risk of coronary heart disease			
Integrase inhibitor	Raltegravir	√	
	Elvitegravir	√	
	Dolutegravir	√	
NRTI*	Tenofovir	√	
	Abacavir		√
Protease inhibitor	Atazanavir/R†	√	
	Darunavir/R†	√	
	Indinavir/R		√
	Lopinavir/R		√
	Fosamprenavir/R		√

*NRTI: nucleoside reverse transcriptase inhibitors (use in combination with either lamivudine or emtricitabine).
†Use in combination with tenofovir/emtricitabine.
ART, antiretroviral therapy; R, ritonavir.

Taken together, elucidating the abacavir/CVD association is probably limited by the fact that studies derived from secondary analyses of RCT data were not appropriately powered to detect increased CHD risk, and that the follow-up may have been too short properly to detect a rare outcome event such as ACS. Furthermore, the observational studies are probably limited by the problem of confounding by indication, because in adjusted analysis where confounding is addressed in these studies, the abacavir/CVD risk association is attenuated. Therefore, use of abacavir should be individualised, taking into consideration the baseline CHD risk.

Overall, conflicting evidence regarding the risk of CHD due to ART may, in part, be related to the study of older cohorts with differences in HIV disease (probably prior severe immunosuppression) and ART (older, more toxic therapies). The much awaited results of the ongoing Strategic Timing of Antiretroviral Treatment (START) trial using newer HIV cohorts with difference HIV disease parameters and ART will provide contemporary clinical and epidemiologic understanding of the association between HIV and CHD. **Figure 5.1** provides a diagrammatic summary of the multiple factors that are likely to contribute to excess risk of CHD among HIV-infected patients.

EVALUATION AND MANAGEMENT OF HIV-ASSOCIATED CHD

CHD risk assessment: limitations of CHD risk prediction rules

In contrast to the general population, where CHD risk prediction equations such as the Framingham risk score are well established and define predicted risk thresholds for initiating specific CHD risk reduction strategies, risk prediction tools have not been formally validated in HIV populations. The Framingham risk score has been shown to underestimate risk when applied to HIV-infected patients [35]. Thus far, the Framingham risk score has not been formally validated for use among HIV-infected patients, but

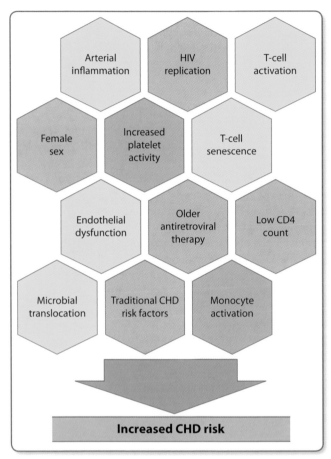

Figure 5.1 Multiple factors that contribute to excess risk of coronary heart disease among HIV-infected patients. Factors in red hexagons have been independently associated with cardiovascular outcomes while those in yellow hexagons have been associated with the presence of subclinical atherosclerosis or are markers of subclinical atherosclerosis among HIV-infected patients. Factors in purple hexagons are hypothesized to contribute to CHD risk.

continues to be used widely in this group. Caution, therefore, needs to be exercised in interpreting lower-risk scores, especially since heart age (i.e. risk for CHD) seems to be higher than real age among HIV-infected patients with lower Framingham risk score. It is notable that the 2013 American College of Cardiology (ACC)/American Heart Association (AHA) risk calculator (Pooled Cohorts Equation), which has been reported to overestimate risk in the general population, has yet to be studied in the setting of HIV.

The use of imaging modalities such as CT-based coronary artery calcium score, carotid intima media thickness, brachial artery flow mediated dilation and, most recently, aortic PET have provided insights into the pathophysiology of HIV-associated CHD risk, but widespread clinical use in CHD risk prediction remains limited, both in the general population and in HIV. There are no clear clinical recommendations for use of these imaging modalities to estimate and manage CHD risk among HIV-infected patients.

Prevention of HIV-associated CHD
Role of ART
Treatment of HIV is a recommended strategy to reduce CVD risk, endorsed by major HIV treatment guidelines. While earlier reports demonstrated associations between individual

ART medications, the decrease in HIV-related inflammation and immune activation that results from HIV treatment and virologic suppression is thought to be significantly more important in decreasing CVD risk. ART is therefore thought to have a net beneficial effect on CVD risk.

Traditional CVD risk factors

Access to cardiac/lipid neutral ART and use of general population CHD prevention strategies [36] are the cornerstone of CHD prevention among HIV-infected patients (**Table 5.2**). Ideally, the cardiologist should work collaboratively with the HIV specialist to develop a comprehensive CHD management strategy.

It is unclear, however, whether general population guidelines on CVD prevention are appropriate in HIV, as the mechanism of HIV-associated CVD differs, and general population guidelines do not reflect the novel, HIV-related inflammation and immune dysfunction thought to underlie the increased risk. Nonetheless, adhering to established guidelines seems likely to be beneficial in the absence of further data and HIV-specific guidelines. Among different HIV populations, there is evidence of suboptimal screening and management of traditional CHD risk factors [37], such as provision of aspirin, lipid lowering agents, antihypertensive treatment and smoking cessation counselling and pharmacotherapy. As stated in the HIV Primary Care Guidelines [38] and European AIDS Clinical Society guidelines [36], lifestyle interventions such as increasing physical activity, smoking cessation and weight management are key in mitigating CHD risk. Smoking cessation has been shown specifically to reduce CVD risk in HIV, and pharmacologic interventions for smoking cessation have been found to be safe. Although several HIV-specific smoking cessation interventions have been tested with varying results, it is recommended to follow general population guidelines and to utilise the frequency of HIV care encounters to provide repeated intensive counseling. Screening for diabetes mellitus is best achieved using fasting glucose. Given that HbA1C may underestimate glycaemia in HIV, lower cutoff values (e.g. 5.8%) may be indicated if used as a screening tool.

Management of cholesterol and statin therapy in HIV-associated CHD

When selecting ART, premorbid dyslipidaemia and overall CHD risk need to be considered in choosing specific medications in the context of baseline CVD risk assessment. The 2014 International Antiviral Society–USA panel recommends against abacavir use, if possible, given the conflicting data regarding CHD risk related to abacavir exposure. Ritonavir-boosted lopinavir, indinavir and fosamprenavir should be avoided, given their strong association with outcome of CHD. Integrase inhibitors and ritonavir-boosted atazanavir or darunavir are preferred for patients with dyslipidaemia or elevated CVD risk because of their neutral effect on lipids.

Dyslipidaemia treatment thresholds should follow general population guidelines. The 2013 ACC/AHA cholesterol guidelines have caused a paradigm shift in cholesterol management, and the extent to which these guidelines should be applied in the setting of HIV – as opposed to using ATP-IIII-based low-density lipoprotein (LDL) cutoffs – remains uncertain. Diet modification among HIV-infected patients with dyslipidaemia is recommended and has been associated with improvement in lipid profiles. Statin and ART drug–drug interaction are common and should always be considered when starting statin therapy. The HIV Primary Care Guidelines provide comprehensive overviews of ART–statin interactions.

When HIV-infected patients on statin therapy develop muscle toxicity and elevations in serum creatine kinase, integrase inhibitor (especially raltegravir) induced myalgias should be considered in the differential in addition to considering statin effects. Recent evidence suggests that while the ezetemibe–fenofibrate combination is well tolerated and can lower total cholesterol, LDL cholesterol and non-HDL cholesterol as effectively as pravastatin, the ezetemibe–fenofibrate combination also had the added benefit of resulting in increases in HDL cholesterol and decreases in triglycerides, both of which are common lipid abnormalities among HIV-infected patients.

SUMMARY

CHD is projected to be the leading cause of mortality, both in resource-limited settings and also globally, by year 2030, with HIV as second and third cause of mortality, globally and in resource-limited settings, respectively. Addressing this double epidemic of CHD and HIV will require cross-disciplinary research and clinical care, given the complex mechanisms that drive excess CHD risk among HIV-infected individuals, including traditional CHD risk factors, immune dysregulation, HIV replication and possible ART toxicity. Screening for CHD risk factors and providing recommended general population interventions to reduce CHD risk among HIV-infected patients should be prioritised and performed with careful attention to the limitations of current CHD risk assessment tools among HIV-infected patients. Additional research on the aetiology, risk assessment and treatment of HIV-associated CHD is needed to address this important complication and improve care for HIV populations.

Key points for clinical practice

- HIV confers an approximate 1.5–2-fold increased risk of CHD.
- The increased risk of CHD observed in HIV-infected patients is not fully explained by traditional CVD risk factors.
- HIV-related inflammation and immune activation appear to be important drivers of increased CVD risk in HIV.
- The applicability of general CVD guidelines is unclear in HIV populations.
- Modification of traditional CVD risk factors is important to prevent CVD in HIV populations.
- Antiretroviral therapy, despite possible proatherogenic effects of individual medications, is thought to reduce CVD risk.
- Managing noncommunicable complications is an increasingly important component of long-term HIV care.

REFERENCES

1. Klein D, Hurley LB, Quesenberry CP Jr, Sidney S. Do protease inhibitors increase the risk for coronary heart disease in patients with HIV-1 infection? J Acquir Immune Defic Syndr 2002; 30:471–477.
2. Currier JS, Taylor A, Boyd F, et al. Coronary heart disease in HIV-infected individuals. J Acquir Immune Defic Syndr 2003; 33:506–512.
3. Triant VA, Lee H, Hadigan C, Grinspoon SK. Increased acute myocardial infarction rates and cardiovascular risk factors among patients with human immunodeficiency virus disease. J Clin Endocrinol Metab 2007; 92:2506–2512.

4. Obel N, Thomsen HF, Kronborg G, et al. Ischemic heart disease in HIV-infected and HIV-uninfected individuals: a population-based cohort study. Clin Infect Dis 2007; 44:1625–1631.

5. Lang S, Mary-Krause M, Cotte L, et al. Increased risk of myocardial infarction in HIV-infected patients in France, relative to the general population. AIDS 2010; 24:1228–1230.

6. Durand M, Sheehy O, Baril JG, Lelorier J, Tremblay CL. Association between HIV infection, antiretroviral therapy, and risk of acute myocardial infarction: a cohort and nested case-control study using Quebec's public health insurance database. J Acquir Immune Defic Syndr 2011; 57:245–253.

7. Freiberg MS, Chang CC, Kuller LH, et al. HIV infection and the risk of acute myocardial infarction. JAMA Intern Med 2013; 173:614–622.

8. Silverberg MJ, Leyden WA, Xu L, et al. Immunodeficiency and risk of myocardial infarction among HIV-positive individuals with access to care. J Acquir Immune Defic Syndr 2014; 65:160–166.

9. Bloomfield GS, Khazanie P, Morris A, et al. HIV and noncommunicable cardiovascular and pulmonary diseases in low- and middle-income countries in the ART era: what we know and best directions for future research. J Acquir Immune Defic Syndr 2014; 67:S40–S53.

10. Freiberg MS, Chang CC, Skanderson M, et al. The risk of incident coronary heart disease among veterans with and without HIV and hepatitis C. Circ Cardiovasc Qual Outcomes 2011; 4:425–432.

11. Syed FF, Sani MU. Recent advances in HIV-associated cardiovascular diseases in Africa. Heart 2013; 99:1146–1153.

12. Heikinheimo T, Chimbayo D, Kumwenda JJ, Kampondeni S, Allain TJ. Stroke outcomes in Malawi, a country with high prevalence of HIV: a prospective follow-up study. PLoS One 2012; 7:e33765.

13. Grinspoon S, Carr A. Cardiovascular risk and body-fat abnormalities in HIV-infected adults. N Engl J Med 2005; 352:48–62.

14. Reinsch N, Neuhaus K, Esser S, et al. Are HIV patients undertreated? Cardiovascular risk factors in HIV: results of the HIV-HEART study. Eur J Prev Cardiol 2012; 19:267–274.

15. Strategies for Management of Antiretroviral Therapy (SMART) Study Group, El-Sadr WM, Lundgren J, et al. CD4+ count-guided interruption of antiretroviral treatment. N Engl J Med 2006; 355:2283–2296.

16. Phillips AN, Carr A, Neuhaus J, et al. Interruption of antiretroviral therapy and risk of cardiovascular disease in persons with HIV-1 infection: exploratory analyses from the SMART trial. Antivir Ther 2008; 13:177–187.

17. Kuller LH, Tracy R, Belloso W, et al. Inflammatory and coagulation biomarkers and mortality in patients with HIV infection. PLoS Med 2008; 5:e203.

18. Hsue PY, Deeks SG, Hunt PW. Immunologic basis of cardiovascular disease in HIV-infected adults. J Infect Dis 2012; 205:S375–S382.

19. Lang S, Mary-Krause M, Simon A, et al. HIV replication and immune status are independent predictors of the risk of myocardial infarction in HIV-infected individuals. Clin Infect Dis 2012; 55:600–607.

20. Triant VA, Regan S, Lee H, et al. Association of immunologic and virologic factors with myocardial infarction rates in a US healthcare system. J Acquir Immune Defic Syndr 2010; 55:615–619.

21. Subramanian S, Tawakol A, Burdo TH, et al. Arterial inflammation in patients with HIV. JAMA 2012; 308:379–386.

22. Lo J, Abbara S, Shturman L, et al. Increased prevalence of subclinical coronary atherosclerosis detected by coronary computed tomography angiography in HIV-infected men. AIDS 2010; 24:243–253.

23. Zanni MV, Abbara S, Lo J, et al. Increased coronary atherosclerotic plaque vulnerability by coronary computed tomography angiography in HIV-infected men. AIDS 2013; 27:1263–1272.

24. Tawakol A, Lo J, Zanni MV, et al. Increased arterial inflammation relates to high-risk coronary plaque morphology in HIV-infected patients. J Acquir Immune Defic Syndr 2014; 66:164–171.

25. Stein JH, Brown TT, Ribaudo HJ, et al. Ultrasonographic measures of cardiovascular disease risk in antiretroviral treatment-naive individuals with HIV infection. AIDS 2013; 27:929–937.

26. Ho JE, Deeks SG, Hecht FM, et al. Initiation of antiretroviral therapy at higher nadir CD4+ T-cell counts is associated with reduced arterial stiffness in HIV-infected individuals. AIDS 2010; 24:1897–1905.

27. Papakonstantinou VD, Chini M, Mangafas N, et al. In vivo effect of two first-line ART regimens on inflammatory mediators in male HIV patients. Lipids Health Dis 2014; 13:90.

28. O'Brien M, Montenont E, Hu L, et al. Aspirin attenuates platelet activation and immune activation in HIV-infected subjects on antiretroviral therapy: a pilot study. J Acquir Immune Defic Syndr 2013; 63:280–288.

29. Thompson MA, Aberg JA, Hoy JF, et al. Antiretroviral treatment of adult HIV infection: 2012 recommendations of the International Antiviral Society-USA panel. JAMA 2012; 308:387–402.

30. DAD Study Group, Friis-Møller N, Reiss P, et al. Class of antiretroviral drugs and the risk of myocardial infarction. N Engl J Med 2007; 356:1723–1735.

31. DAD Study Group, Sabin CA, Worm SW, et al. Use of nucleoside reverse transcriptase inhibitors and risk of myocardial infarction in HIV-infected patients enrolled in the D:A:D study: a multi-cohort collaboration. Lancet 2008; 371:1417–1426.

32. Ding X, Andraca-Carrera E, Cooper C, et al. No association of abacavir use with myocardial infarction: findings of an FDA meta-analysis. J Acquir Immune Defic Syndr 2012; 61:441–447.

33. Monforte A, Reiss P, Ryom L, et al. Atazanavir is not associated with an increased risk of cardio or cerebrovascular disease events. AIDS 2013; 27:407–415.

34. Ribaudo HJ, Benson CA, Zheng Y, et al. No risk of myocardial infarction associated with initial antiretroviral treatment containing abacavir: short and long-term results from ACTG A5001/ALLRT. Clin Infect Dis 2011; 52:929–940.

35. Law MG, Friis-Møller N, El-Sadr WM, et al. The use of the Framingham equation to predict myocardial infarctions in HIV-infected patients: comparison with observed events in the D:A:D Study. HIV Med 2006; 7:218–230.

36. Lundgren JD, Battegay M, Behrens G, et al. European AIDS Clinical Society (EACS) guidelines on the prevention and management of metabolic diseases in HIV. HIV Med 2008; 9:72–81.

37. Lichtenstein KA, Armon C, Buchacz K, et al. Provider compliance with guidelines for management of cardiovascular risk in HIV-infected patients. Prev Chronic Dis 2013; 10:E10.

38. Aberg JA, Gallant JE, Ghanem KG, et al. Primary care guidelines for the management of persons infected with HIV: 2013 update by the HIV Medicine Association of the Infectious Diseases Society of America. Clin Infect Dis 2014; 58:1–10.

Chapter 6

Percutaneous valve intervention

Thomas M Snow, Philip MacCarthy

INTRODUCTION

As the global population has aged, the incidence of degenerative valve disease has increased. Calcific aortic stenosis and mitral insufficiency are common and convey significant morbidity and mortality. Transcatheter intervention has evolved in a field where valve disease was previously treatable only with conventional surgery or medical management. Contemporary technology now offers hope to individuals with acquired valve dysfunction and prohibitive or high surgical risk. It offers minimally invasive therapy that has been demonstrated to not only improve symptoms and quality of life but also prevent recurrent hospital admissions and, in some cases, increase life expectancy.

Research and development in this field, supported both academically and in the commercial sector, has refined devices, with many of the aortic prostheses now in their third or fourth iteration. Miniaturised delivery systems, and increased operator knowledge and expertise have reduced procedure times and complication rates, and therefore shortened hospital admissions.

Over the last 12 years, the field of transcatheter intervention for structural heart disease has developed at an unprecedented rate. There are now treatment options for all four heart valves, with the aortic and mitral valves being the main focus of development, but with potential to expand into the fields of pulmonary and tricuspid intervention.

This chapter outlines the current state of both commercially available percutaneous valve systems and areas of ongoing research and development.

AORTIC VALVE

Aortic stenosis

Aortic stenosis is common in elderly patients – perhaps more common than was originally thought. The Euro-Heart survey indicated a prevalence of 2–7% of the general population over 65 years of age [1]. Once symptomatic, it carries a very poor prognosis when left untreated with a mortality of 50% at 2 years, a figure that has not changed for decades [2]. Several studies have shown that many of these patients were not being offered surgical valve replacement, assessed by an expert 'Heart Team'.

Thomas M Snow BSc MBBCh MPhil MRCP, Department of Cardiology, King's College Hospital, London, UK

Philip MacCarthy BSc MBChB PhD FRCP, Department of Cardiology, King's College Hospital, London, UK. Email: philip.maccarthy@nhs.net (for correspondence)

It is more than a decade since Professor Alain Cribier's 'first-in-man' percutaneous aortic valve implantation (transcatheter aortic valve implantation, TAVI) [3]. Before this pivotal case, the treatment of severe symptomatic aortic stenosis in patients with high or prohibitive surgical risk was limited to medical management, with or without balloon aortic valvuloplasty (BAV) [4,5]. The latter, while still performed, often as a bridge to definitive treatment or to allow assessment of symptomatic improvement, confers little improvement in prognosis.

Alain Cribier first implanted a bovine pericardial, trileaflet TAVI valve sewn inside a balloon expandable stent via an anterograde, trans-septal approach. The anterograde approach was problematic; and it was John Webb et al who successfully developed a method of delivering the valve prosthesis retrogradely via the femoral/iliac artery [6].

Early devices had several acknowledged weaknesses. There were high rates of bleeding/vascular complications from access sites due to the large calibre delivery systems and unacceptable rates of paravalvar regurgitation, often due to the great variability of both anatomy and distribution of calcium on the valve leaflets and annulus. Rates of permanent pacemaker (PPM) implantation were also high (particularly in the CoreValve group). Nevertheless, despite these limitations, an impressive evidence base emerged as the procedure became more widespread.

The traditional on-label indication for TAVI is for severe symptomatic aortic stenosis of a trileaflet valve, in a patient deemed unfit or high risk for conventional surgical aortic valve replacement. TAVI has been demonstrated as superior to medical therapy (± BAV–PARTNER trial) [7] and at least noninferior to high-risk conventional surgical aortic valve replacement (PARTNER A) [8] and the recent CoreValve PIVOTAL Trial [9].

As a result of this success, more than 150,000 percutaneous aortic valves have now been implanted worldwide, with rapid expansion particularly in Europe and more latterly in the USA.

Miniaturisation of vascular access sheaths and delivery systems, from the early 22Fr devices to the latest 14/16Fr devices has reduced vascular complication rates and facilitated fully percutaneous procedures in contrast to surgical femoral arterial closure. Such evolution of the technique has prompted operators to perform TAVI without general anaesthesia (using conscious sedation alone) and has also enabled earlier mobilisation, which is undoubtedly beneficial, both for the patient and the TAVI centre.

Alternative vascular access via the subclavian, axillary and carotid arteries has been used in certain patient groups. The surgical transapical and transaortic approaches are possible where anatomy prohibits the more conventional peripheral approach.

Technological advances in TAVI have been rapid with the first-generation devices (the Medtronic CoreValve and Edwards Sapien systems) being the first to demonstrate improved clinical outcomes over the mid-to-long term. Concerns over valve durability appear unfounded and the earliest valves, having been implanted 8–10 years ago, demonstrate excellent ongoing haemodynamic performance.

The current generation devices, as outlined below (**Table 6.1**), are now available across a broader range of valve sizes, have reduced the incidence and severity of paravalvar insufficiency, are more predictable during deployment and, in some, can be retrieved or repositioned in a manner that was not previously possible.

Currently used valve prostheses

Sapien (Edwards Lifesciences Corp, USA)

The Sapien XT prosthesis (**Figure 6.1**) is still widely used but the Sapien 3 is an encouraging development. This fourth-generation valve from Edwards, based on the original Cribier–

Table 6.1 Aortic valve technology: CE-marked and non-CE-marked devices			
Device (manufacturer)	Mechanism of deployment	Access route	Treatable aortic annulus size (mm)
CoreValve Evolut R (Medtronic Inc.)	Self-expanding nitinol frame	Transfemoral, trans-subclavian [14F (true outer 18F)]	18–30
Sapien XT (Edwards Lifesciences)	Balloon expandable	Transfemoral + transapical (24F)	18–27
Sapien 3 (Edwards Lifesciences)	Balloon expandable	Transfemoral (14–16F) transapical (18–21F)	18–28 (TOE) 20.5–29.5 (MDCT)
Lotus Valve (Boston Scientific)	Braided nitinol wire mechanically expanded on implantation	Transfemoral (18–20F)	19–27
Direct Flow (Direct Flow Medical)	Aortic and ventricular 'inflatable' rings with strut framework	Transfemoral (18F)	19–28
JenaValve (JenaValve)	Porcine aortic root sewn into a nitinol external frame – self-expanding	Transapical (32F) transfemoral (18F)	21–27
Engager (Medtronic Inc.)	Self-expanding nitinol frame with support 'arms'	Transapical/transaortic (29F)	21–26.7
Acurate TA (Symetis)	Self-expanding nitinol frame	Transapical (28F sheathless)	21–27
Portico (St Jude Medical)	Self-expanding nitinol frame	Transfemoral (18F) transpical (24F sheathless)	19–21

MDCT, multi-detector CT; TOE, transoesophageal echo.

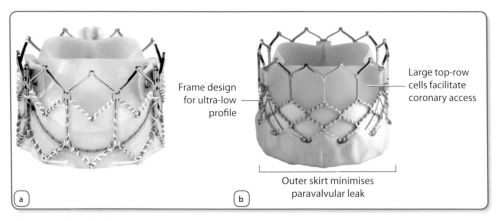

Frame design for ultra-low profile

Large top-row cells facilitate coronary access

Outer skirt minimises paravalvular leak

a   b

Figure 6.1 Edwards Lifescience transcatheter heart valves. (a) Sapien XT valve. (b) Sapien 3 valve. With permission from Edwards Lifesciences, Irvine, CA, USA.

Edwards valve, uses a balloon expandable framework within which a bovine pericardial trileaflet valve is sewn. Aortic valve annuli between 18 and 28 mm (transoesophageal echo (TOE) sizing) or 20.5–29.5 mm [multidetector CT (MDCT) sizing] can be accommodated using this valve system. The inner 'skirt' has been continued with the addition of an external skirt at the inflow, to further improve sealing in the native annulus and minimise paravalvular leak.

There has been a marked reduction in the valve delivery system profile to 14Fr in the 23–26 mm valve sizes, with an increment to 16Fr for those larger valves (29 mm). This should not only reduce vascular complication rates, but also allow use of this system in patients with smaller calibre ileofemoral vessels (>5.5 mm). A further reduction in both sizing and profile has been seen for the transapical Certitude delivery system (21Fr from 24Fr with the earlier generation ASCENDRA system).

CoreValve Evolut R (Medtronic, USA)

This newest iteration from Medtronic continues to use a selfexpanding nitinol frame (be it 10 mm shorter than its predecessor) and bovine pericardial valve leaflets (**Figure 6.2**). Alterations to the stent structure have improved deliverability and stability at the level of the left ventricular outflow tract (LVOT), annulus and aortic root. More predictable radial force aids stability in the LVOT and aortic root, while at the level of the neoannulus it is constrained to ensure optimal coronary flow and circularise the neoannulus independent of the native anatomy. An extension of the valve skirt has been designed to further reduce the incidence of paravalvular insufficiency.

There is an extended size range (23, 26, 29 and 32) covering aortic valve annuli from 18 to 30 mm.

Lotus (Boston Scientific Corp, USA)

This valve is designed from a single-braided nitinol wire that houses a trileaflet bovine pericardial valve and is available in three valve sizes with an effective annular range of 19–27 mm (**Figure 6.3**). The valve itself is extended for delivery, to a length of 70 mm and is then shortened manually to 19 mm with radial expansion on deployment. An overlying Adaptive seal sleeve is present; improving paravalvular apposition even in heavily calcified valves thus reducing the risk of regurgitation. The valve can be unsheathed and resheathed prior to deployment to aid positioning and retrievability and a separate releasing knob on the delivery system finalises deployment once the operator is content.

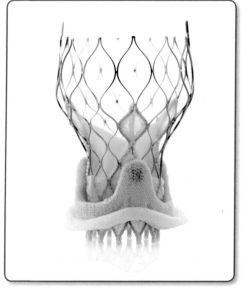

Figure 6.2 CoreValve Evolut R implanted in a surgical bioprosthesis (valve-in-valve). With permission from Medtronic Inc., Minneapolis, MN, USA.

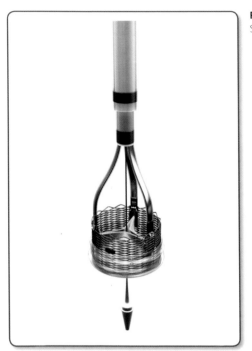

Figure 6.3 Lotus Valve. With permission from Boston Scientific, Natick, MA, USA.

Direct Flow (Direct Flow Medical Inc, USA)

This is a trileaflet, bovine pericardial valve sewn into a nonmetallic framework composed of struts supporting an inflow (ventricular) manually inflated ring and outflow (aortic) ring. Positioned initially in the ventricle, this valve is retracted into position (transfemoral approach), guided by TOE/ fluoroscopy. When optimally sited, the inflow ring is inflated and this process is repeated for the aortic ring, thereby securing the valve within the native valve annulus. Valve gradients and regurgitation can be assessed throughout the process to ensure acceptable haemodynamics.

Delivery is through a fully sheathed 18Fr system that can treat aortic annuli from 19 to 28 mm.

Other devices

There are a number of other devices which are used in various centres and are building an evidence base in registries and small clinical trials.

JenaValve (JenaValve Technology GmbH, Germany)

The only transcatheter valve CE marked for both severe native aortic stenosis and regurgitation (the latter since 2013) uses a porcine aortic root covered externally by a porcine pericardial skirt, which is then sewn into a nitinol external frame. This valve has three so-called feelers which are released in the aortic root and orientated by the operator to engage the coronary sinuses (CSs), thereby ensuring correct valve positioning and minimising the risk of coronary compromise.

A transfemoral version was released last year and is delivered by an 18Fr catheter system.

Acurate TA (Symetis SA, Switzerland)

Designed for the transapical approach (28Fr sheathless) this porcine valve is mounted inside a nitinol frame. It also uses an internal skirt to minimise paravalvular insufficiency and is fully retrievable up to the point after compression of the native valve leaflets. A transfemoral version, the Acurate neo is delivered via an 18Fr delivery system.

Engager (Medtronic Inc, USA)

Delivered via a transapical or direct aortic approach, this selfexpanding nitinol stent uses support arms to improve stability in the aortic root by their positioning in the sinuses of valsalva, which may enable the use of this device for aortic regurgitation as well as aortic stenosis.

Delivery requires a larger 29F introducer and its use is therefore limited to central access.

Expanding indications

Novel off-label indications now include transcatheter intervention in intermediate surgical risk patients. Whether TAVI is appropriate in lower-risk patient populations will depend on whether the current limitations of the technique can be overcome, namely paravalvar leak, pacemaker requirement, vascular injury and stroke risk. Initially, there were concerns about valve prosthesis durability, but experience to date suggests that TAVI valve prostheses last as long as surgical bioprostheses. The appropriateness of a move into a lower-risk population will be better defined by ongoing randomised trials comparing the techniques in these patients, including UK TAVI, SURTAVI and PARTNER 2. These trials will also yield important information about cost-effectiveness, which will clearly influence the growth of transcatheter techniques.

Other newer indications include the treatment of the bicuspid aortic valve, which has traditionally been thought to be less suitable for TAVI due to asymmetric anatomy/calcification, often a very oval annulus and coexistent aortic root disease. An important distinction needs to be made between the congenitally bicuspid valve and a degenerate, calcified tricuspid valve, which has undergone fusion of the cusps in the disease process – the so-called functionally bicuspid valve. Early studies of TAVI in bicuspid valves have been published [10] and have shown that although possible, results are not as good, particularly in terms of the rates of paravalvar AR post-TAVI. Most operators agree that each patient and valve anatomy need to be assessed carefully by the Heart Team, taking these issues in to account.

Aortic regurgitation

Transcatheter therapy for pure aortic regurgitation is more challenging because of the lack of calcification around the valve to anchor the prosthesis in this pathology. Moreover, aortic regurgitation is often associated with dilatation/disease of the aortic root. However, some of the newer devices have aortic cusp clipping systems [e.g. the JenaValve and Engager (see above)], which allow effective treatment of this anatomy.

Failing bioprosthetic aortic valves

It has long been appreciated that transcatheter valve therapy is a potentially excellent treatment for failing bioprostheses [11,12] and homograft aortic roots [13] to the extent that surgical practice has changed and bioprostheses are being implanted in younger patients with an expectation that they can have a valve-in-valve procedure when the surgical valve fails. The technique has advantages in that often, the annulus (i.e. the sewing ring of the surgical prosthesis) is easily seen radiographically, there is (usually with most surgical valves) less risk of coronary ostial occlusion and a lower risk of new pacemaker requirement.

Early data emerging from a multinational registry of 459 patients suggest that TAVI in a degenerative surgical bioprosthesis can yield acceptable survival rates at 1 year (83.2%). Smaller bioprostheses (<21 mm) and surgical valve stenosis were markers of lower survival in this cohort [14]. This indication is now well established and more data will guide its use in the coming years.

MITRAL VALVE

Mitral stenosis

The commonest aetiology for acquired mitral valve stenosis, rheumatic heart disease, is associated with significant morbidity and mortality and is now relatively uncommon in first-world countries. Unfortunately, it remains a significant problem in developing countries.

European guidelines for the management of mitral valve stenosis suggest echocardiography as the mainstay for both its diagnosis and surveillance. Treatment strategy is defined by both symptoms (timing of intervention) and valve morphology (percutaneous vs. surgical). Severe mitral stenosis, defined as a mitral valve area <1.5 cm^2 with associated symptoms and favourable valve anatomy is preferentially treated in the first instance with percutaneous mitral commissurotomy. About 80% of patients treated with this approach will achieve a significant increase in mitral valve area (>1.5 cm) and no mitral regurgitation (MR) >2/4 [15]. Follow-up data suggest excellent late efficacy with event-free survival of 30–70% after 10–20 years [16]. Percutaneous treatment is also recommended in those patients with less favourable anatomical characteristics [e.g. calcification of mitral valve of any extent as assessed by fluoroscopy, very small mitral valve area and severe tricuspid regurgitation (TR)], where surgical risk is deemed prohibitive or very high.

Mitral regurgitation

If left untreated, severe degenerative and functional mitral regurgitation (MR) inevitably leads to volume overload and heart failure with debilitating symptoms and often, recurrent hospital admissions. It also carries a poor mid-to-long-term prognosis. Whether driven by ischaemic heart disease, adverse left ventricular remodelling or as a consequence of chordal rupture, myxomatous degeneration of the mitral valve leaflets or calcification, mitral insufficiency is common in elderly patients. Surgical approaches to preserve native valve structure, utilising neochordae, quadrangular resection and annuloplasty rings can now achieve excellent rates of valve repair (as opposed to replacement). It is known that valve repair confers better long-term clinical outcomes than mitral valve replacement, whether bioprosthetic or metallic [17].

In the elderly patient with extensive comorbidity treatment options are often limited to medical management. This involves the optimisation of neurohormonal agents and the judicious use of diuretics to improve symptoms and slow progression of left ventricular (LV) remodelling.

Defined as either primary or secondary, MR is the second commonest valve disease (after aortic stenosis) encountered in everyday practice. Primary MR describes pathology affecting one or more of the components of the mitral valve apparatus. Secondary MR, or functional MR, is defined as valve insufficiency as a consequence of changes to left atrial and/ or ventricular geometry leading to the distortion of an anatomically normal valve. This may be the consequence of coronary artery disease, nonischaemic cardiomyopathy, pressure overload from severe aortic stenosis or volume overload from concomitant aortic regurgitation. As such, treatment may focus on the underlying aetiology, the restoration of valve geometry or a combination of both [18]. Surprisingly, there is still no convincing data that isolated correction of functional MR does any good, either in terms of symptom relief or prognosis. This remains fundamental to understanding the role of the percutaneous mitral valve interventions (**Table 6.2**). Paradoxically, functional MR is technically easier to address percutaneously, yet more clinical gain may be achieved by correcting degenerative MR.

Current transcatheter techniques for treating mitral regurgitation
Leaflet plication
Professor Ottavio Alfieri (Ospedale San Raffaele, Milan, Italy) developed a single-stitch (Alfieri stitch) approach to mitral valve repair, the so-called 'double-orifice' technique, which achieved acceptable short-to-mid-term results without the need for prolonged reconstruction of valve morphology [19]. It is this technique which is mimicked by the leading percutaneous approach to MR, the MitraClip (**Figure 6.4**; Abbott Vascular, CA,

Table 6.2 Mitral valve technology: CE-marked and devices under investigation at the current time		
Site of action	Device	Mechanism of action: current status
Leaflet plication		
	MitraClip	EVEREST I + II clinical trials: CE marked
Space occupier	Mitra-Spacer	Leaflet space occupier: trial stage of development
Annulus		
Indirect annuloplasty	MONARC	Via coronary sinus: discontinued
	CARILLON	Via coronary sinus: TITAN I and II trials
Direct annuloplasty	QuantumCor	Radiofrequency mediated: ongoing development under ValveCure LLC, CA, USA as MitraTight
	ReCor	Ultrasound energy mediated: discontinued
	Mitralign	'Purse-string' mediated: completed clinical trial (results pending)
	Accucinch	'Purse-string' mediated: ongoing development
Chordae		
	MitraFlex	Transapical: ongoing development
	NeoChord	Transpical: ongoing development of NeoChord DS1000 device
LV remodelling		
	iCoapsys	Proof of concept: discontinued.
	VenTouch	External LV saline 'jacket': ongoing development
MV implantation		
	CardiAQ	Antegrade, transeptal: 'First-in-man' implant 2012
LV, left ventriclular; MV, mitral valve.		

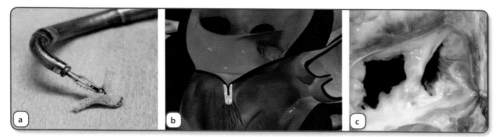

Figure 6.4 MitraClip (Abbott Vascular, CA, USA). (a) Gripper arms retracted prior to deployment. (b) Illustration of MitraClip in-situ with edge-to-edge leaflet plication. (c) Anatomical view of 'double-orifice' valve achieved with MitraClip implantation. With permission from Chiam and Ruiz (2011).

USA). This apposes the anterior and posterior mitral valve leaflets creating a double valve orifice, increasing leaflet coaptation and consequently reducing MR.

Delivered via a transeptal puncture, the delivery system is introduced into the left ventricle via the mitral valve orifice, and the two arms of the clip grip the anterior and posterior valve leaflets under TOE guidance. TOE imaging can then define the extent to which MR has been reduced and can exclude haemodynamically significant iatrogenic mitral valve stenosis. Often more than one clip is deployed to achieve an optimal result [20].

The Endovascular Valve Edge-to-edge Repair Study (EVEREST) I demonstrated the safety and feasibility of this technique with procedural success (defined as a reduction in MR to ≤2+) achieved in 74%. At 12-month freedom from death, mitral valve surgery or MR >2+ was 66% [21].

The follow-on EVEREST II study [22], comparing surgical mitral valve repair with the MitraClip, in 279 patients with severe MR or asymptomatic severe MR with LV dysfunction demonstrated no significant difference in moderate–severe/severe MR and mortality at 4 years, but a higher rate of surgical reoperation for residual MR particularly in the first 12 months (20.4% vs. 2.2%, $P < 0.001$ at 1 year) in patients undergoing percutaneous treatment.

Leaflet space occupier

Developed by Cardiosolutions (Stoughton, MA, USA), the Percu-Pro and Mitra-Spacer device is a polyurethane–silicone buoy that is anchored in the LV apex and positioned in the mitral orifice, thus reducing insufficiency by a reduction in the effective regurgitant orifice area and providing a surface for leaflet apposition at the point of insufficiency. This technology is, as with the MitraClip, associated with the risk of iatrogenic mitral stenosis. Currently, it is in the trial stage of development.

Annular modification – indirect annuloplasty

Mitral valve annuloplasty is a common adjunct in the surgical repair of degenerative mitral valves and often the only intervention required in secondary mitral insufficiency. It seems intuitive, therefore, that percutaneous approaches to achieve the same goal (i.e. a reduction in annular dilatation) may be effective in treating MR via a transcatheter approach.

The MONARC (Edwards Lifesciences, Irvine, CA, USA), VIACOR percutaneous transvenous mitral annuloplasty device (Viacor, Wilmington, MA, USA) and CARILLON mitral contour system (Cardiac Dimensions, Kirkland, WA, USA) access the CS (coronary sinus) via a transvenous approach in an attempt to remodel the mitral valve annulus using a series of anchors within the CS and a cinching mechanism to deflect forward the posterior mitral valve annulus, thereby reducing the dimensions of the mitral valve orifice. There are major limitations with such devices; namely, inconsistency in the degree of posterior mitral annular displacement and therefore reduction in MR and variability in CS anatomy. There is also a risk of coronary artery compression. The presence of an LV lead for cardiac resynchronisation precludes such an approach. Initial trial results have been disappointing and only the latter device has continued in its development.

Annular modification – direct annuloplasty

This is achieved by the directed application of radiofrequency (QuantumCor: Lake Forest, CA, USA) or ultrasound energy (ReCor: Paris, France) to the posterior mitral valve annulus resulting in the heating of annular tissue. Such tissue damage leads to fibrosis and retraction of the posterior mitral valve annulus, hence a proposed reduction in MR. This technology has been limited by the imprecise nature in which energy can be applied, the heterogeneity of the tissues response to energy mediated damage and also the risk of unpredictable results with either mitral stenosis or an inadequate reduction in MR. There are also the potential risks of damage to adjacent structures if energy cannot be accurately applied.

Direct annuloplasty can also be achieved through the implantation of anchors between the anterior and posterior commisures along the posterior LV wall/annulus behind the mitral valve apparatus. Application of tension to this system causes a 'purse-string' effect, which leads to anterior displacement of the posterior wall/annulus and an effective partial (incomplete) annuloplasty. This approach is seen in the Mitralign device (Mitralign, USA) and Accucinch Annuloplasty System (**Figure 6.5**; Guided Delivery Systems, USA).

Chordal implantation

Implanted via a transapical or transeptal approach, these neochordae are anchored both to the LV endocardium and mitral valve leaflets, resulting in a reduction in MR by improving valve coaptation and treatment of leaflet prolapse (MitraFlex: TransCardiac Therapeutics, USA; NeoChord: Neochord Inc. USA).

Left ventricular remodelling

Secondary MR is often a consequence of adverse LV remodelling from both ischaemic and nonischaemic cardiomyopathy. Percutaneous techniques have been developed in

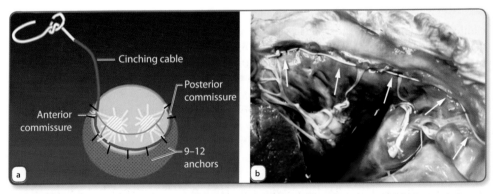

Figure 6.5 Accucinch annuloplasty system. (a) Diagrammatic representation of system action. (b) Anatomical specimen following device deployment in an animal model (arrows denoting suture around posterior mitral valve annulus). With permission from Chiam and Ruiz (2011).

an attempt to achieve positive LV remodelling, thereby restoring geometry and reducing papillary muscle displacement and, therefore, MR. These approaches are more invasive than true transcatheter approaches as they require access to the pericardial space via a mini-thoracotomy. Development continues; early data have been obtained from the now discontinued iCoapsys system (Edwards Lifesciences) and VenTouch system; a saline filled external LV jacket that can be selectively filled to restore LV geometry (Mardil Medical, USA).

Percutaneous mitral valve implantation

This is a new frontier for the treatment of native structural heart disease and an area of intense interest. However, the mitral valve (MV) is functionally and anatomically much more complex than the aortic valve, and the process of fully percutaneous MV replacement has proved challenging.

The CardiAQ (CardiAQ Valve Technologies, Irvine, CA, USA) prosthesis is implanted via an antegrade, transeptal approach. It aims to overcome the inherent difficulties associated with implantation in the mitral position where there is little tissue for apposition and stability, great risk associated with excessive radial force in an elastic and often poorly calcified annulus and further risk in valve positioning where LV outflow could be compromised. This valve remains in development, with the 'first-in-man' implant performed in Copenhagen in 2012.

The first-in-human implants of the Edwards Lifesciences FORTIS valve have been conducted in 2014 but data on this patient cohort have not yet been published.

All of these technologies are yet to reach large-scale trials and remain in the early stages of development.

There have been many documented cases of mitral insufficiency due to a 'failing' mitral bioprosthesis or mitral annuloplasty ring being treated successfully with the Edwards Sapien transcatheter aortic valve [23,24] – 'valve-in-valve' or 'valve-in-ring' therapy in the mitral position. Excellent haemodynamic results have been reported, with the trileaflet aortic prosthesis deployed within the surgical bioprosthesis or annuloplasty ring. Similar 'valve-in-valve' procedures have been reported for stenosed mitral surgical prostheses, again with good outcomes. Such techniques can be performed via the transapical approach or femoral, transvenous approach (across the interatrial septum), although the latter is technically challenging with the current delivery systems.

PULMONARY VALVE

Clinical experience in the treatment of patients, both children and adults, with 'failing' right ventricular outflow tract (RVOT) conduits (>16 mm in diameter when first implanted), both regurgitant and stenotic, has been with the Melody Transcatheter Pulmonary Valve (**Figure 6.6**) system (Medtronic, Minneapolis, MN, USA). This is a balloon expandable system with a trileaflet, pericardial valve sewn into a stent and delivered via a 22Fr delivery system. Studies have been limited in both this group and a smaller group of patients with native, nonconduit RVOT obstruction [25].

TRICUSPID VALVE

As with the pulmonary valve, there is limited clinical experience in the transcatheter treatment of tricuspid valve disease. There are a number of published case reports of the use of the balloon expandable Edwards Sapien valve prosthesis in the tricuspid position for

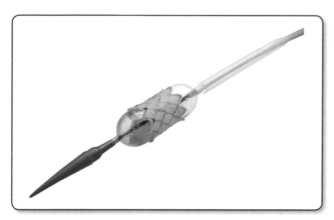

Figure 6.6 Melody valve. With permission from Medtronic Inc., Minneapolis, MN, USA.

the treatment of both TR and stenosis in degenerate bioprostheses [26,27]. These results are promising; however, there remains little evidence for their use in degenerative native valves. There are as yet only individual case reports of custom-made transcatheter valves implanted at the cavoatrial junction in patients with severe TR and right heart failure with prohibitive surgical risk [28].

The Medtronic Melody valve, designed for implantation in the pulmonary/ RVOT position, has also been successfully implanted in both failing bioprosthetic tricuspid and MV s as an off-label indication [29].

ADVANCES IN IMAGING TECHNOLOGY

Advances in imaging technology, particularly in three-dimensional (3D) echocardiography and CT techniques, have underpinned the evolution of transcatheter therapy. Preoperative planning has become increasingly sophisticated with accurate aortic annulus sizing, estimations of prosthesis size needed to 'circularise' an oval aortic annulus, detailed mapping of eccentric valve calcification and analysis of important anatomical relationships (e.g. the distance of coronary ostia from the aortic valves). This has enabled precise tailoring of prostheses to native anatomy and reduced complications such as paravalvar aortic regurgitation, coronary obstruction and annular rupture. Periprocedural 3D TOE has also facilitated valve deployment, rapid identification of complications and 'online' evaluation of paravalvar aortic regurgitation, thus guiding the need for postdilatation of implanted prostheses.

As transcatheter valve techniques become more sophisticated and with more involvement of the MV, the need for improved imaging will only increase.

THE IMPORTANCE OF THE 'HEART TEAM'

Perhaps the most important legacy of the TAVI revolution has been the Heart Team. Every TAVI centre now has a multidisciplinary group of clinicians (interventional cardiologists, cardiothoracic surgeons, cardiac anaesthetists, imaging specialists and care of the elderly physicians) that assesses the clinical scenario, cardiac and noncardiac co-morbidity and vascular/valvular anatomy of each patient. When successful, this allows specific therapy to be tailored to individual patients, whether it is medical, surgical or transcatheter in nature.

The advent of the Heart Team has encouraged a culture of early identification and investigation of valvular heart disease in referring physicians, thus exposing patients to expert opinion earlier in their natural history. It has also focussed clinicians' minds on issues such as accurate aortic annulus sizing and the importance of paravalvar AR, which were not always adequately appreciated before the era of transcatheter valve therapy. In addition, the Heart Team approach has fostered teamwork and shared responsibility, which has had a major beneficial effect on patient care.

CONCLUSION – FUTURE VISION

Transcatheter valve intervention has evolved at a rapid rate over the last decade. There has been great interest in minimally invasive valve intervention both from the perspective of the patient and healthcare professionals, who are now able to offer treatments for disease that previously conveyed a dismal prognosis. Research and development of both new valve designs and evolution of existing devices and delivery systems aim to offer new therapies for these previously unmet needs.

Severe symptomatic aortic stenosis and its treatment with transcatheter technology is now widely accepted as optimal therapy in patients unable to undergo conventional surgical valve replacement. Whether such technology should be offered to lower-risk patients remains to be seen and is perhaps the biggest question currently being addressed by clinical trials. The management of concomitant coronary artery disease, minimising paravalvar regurgitation, reducing PPM implantation rates and the incidence of

Table 6.3 Current issues for further research and development in transcatheter aortic valve implantation	
Technical issue	**Ongoing research/ proposed solution**
Vascular complications/ bleeding	Miniaturisation of valve delivery systems Alternative access routes (e.g. transaortic) Increased operator expertise and improved vascular closure devices (e.g. Perclose ProGlide suture-mediated closure system – Abbott Vascular, CA, USA)
PPM implantation	Rates variable between valve type – CoreValve (higher valve implantation to prevent compression of the infra-nodal conduction tissue) Guidelines for PPM implantation following TAVI Attention to higher valve placement
Acute kidney injury	Reduced contrast burden Reduced haemodynamic disturbance – reduce rapid pacing by avoiding BAV Embolic protection devices
Cerebrovascular events	Embolic protection devices TAVI performed without preceding BAV to minimise valve manipulation
Valve sizing	Use of multimodality imaging MDCT vs. 3D TOE
Paravalvar regurgitation	Valve 'skirt' and 'seal' designs Accurate valve sizing
Management of concomitant coronary artery disease	Meta-analyses and registry data suggest a conservative approach guided by the Heart Team is optimal Ongoing ACTIVATION Clinical Trial (UK based) randomising patients to PCI or medical management prior to TAVI

3D, three-dimensional; BAV, balloon aortic valvuloplasty; MDCT, multi-detector CT; PPM, Permanent pacemaker; TAVI, transcatheter aortic valve implantation; TOE, transoesophageal echo.

periprocedural acute kidney injury and cerebrovascular events are all issues that remain areas of great research activity (**Table 6.3**).

As our understanding of transcatheter technology and technical expertise at performing such procedures improves, we are likely to see advances into new areas and lower-risk patient groups. It is possible that we may see treatment options for a majority of heart valve disease in the next 10–20 years; however, which patients are best served by such an approach remains unclear. The hybrid surgical and transcatheter approach may well develop further to meet such demand being guided by the most important component of this new therapy, the Heart Team.

Key points for clinical practice

- TAVI is widely accepted as the preferred treatment for symptomatic severe aortic stenosis and high surgical risk.
- The refinement of valve prostheses and their delivery systems have reduced complication rates and broadened the anatomical range treatable with TAVI.
- Ongoing clinical trials are reviewing the use of TAVI in lower surgical risk patients.
- 'Off-label' indications for TAVI include the treatment of degenerate bioprostheses, native aortic valve insufficiency and transcatheter aortic valves in nonaortic positions (e.g. failing mitral bioprostheses).
- Advances in the percutaneous treatment of MR now offer adjuncts to optimal medical management in patients with comorbidities precluding conventional surgery.
- MV intervention is in its infancy with the MitraClip the only CE-marked device.
- Novel approaches to both primary and secondary MR are in development.
- Right ventricular outflow and tricuspid valve percutaneous intervention is likely to develop further as aortic valve technology is adapted for use in nonaortic positions.

REFERENCES

1. Iung B, Baron G, Butchart EG, et al. A prospective survey of patients with valvular heart disease in Europe: the Euro Heart Survey on Valvular Heart Disease. Eur Heart J 2003; 24:1231–1243.
2. Lester SJ, Heilbron B, Gin K, et al. The natural history and rate of progression of aortic stenosis. Chest 1998; 113:1109–1114.
3. Cribier A, Eltchaninoff H, Bash A, et al. Percutaneous transcatheter implantation of an aortic valve prosthesis for calcific aortic stenosis: first human case description. Circulation 2002; 106:3006–3008.
4. Serruys PW, Luijten HE, Beatt KJ, et al. Percutaneous balloon valvuloplasty for calcific aortic stenosis. A treatment 'sine cure'? Eur Heart J 1988; 9:782–794.
5. Daly MJ, Monaghan M, Hamilton A, et al. Short-term efficacy of palliative balloon aortic valvuloplasty in selected patients with high operative risk. J Invasive Cardiol 2012; 24:58–62.
6. Webb JG, Pasupati S, Humphries K, et al. Percutaneous transarterial aortic valve replacement in selected high-risk patients with aortic stenosis. Circulation 2007; 116:755–763.
7. Leon MB, Smith CR, Mack M, et al. Transcatheter aortic-valve implantation for aortic stenosis in patients who cannot undergo surgery. N Engl J Med 2010; 363:1597–1607.
8. Smith CR, Leon MB, Mack MJ, et al. Transcatheter versus surgical aortic-valve replacement in high-risk patients. N Engl J Med 2011; 364:2187–2198.
9. Adams D, Popma JJ, Reardon MJ, et al. Transcatheter aortic-valve replacement with a self-expanding prosthesis. N Engl J Med 2014; 370:1790–1798.
10. Yousef A, Simard T, Pourdjabbar A, et al. Performance of transcatheter aortic valve implantation in patients with bicuspid aortic valve: systematic review. Int J Cardiol 2014; 176:562–564.

11. Piazza N, Bleiziffer S, Brockmann G, et al. Transcatheter aortic valve implantation for failing surgical aortic bioprosthetic valve: from concept to clinical application and evaluation. JACC Cardiovasc Interv 2011; 4:721–742.

12. Wenaweser P, Buellesfeld L, Gerckens U, Grube E. Percutaneous aortic valve replacement for severe aortic regurgitation in degenerated bioprosthesis: the first valve-in-valve procedure using the Corevalve Revalving system. Catheter Cardiovasc Interv 2007; 70:760–764.

13. Chan PH, Di Mario C, Davies SW, et al. Transcatheter aortic valve implantation in degenerate failing aortic homograft root replacements. J Am Coll Cardiol 2011; 58:1729–1730.

14. Dvir D, Webb JG, Bleiziffer S, et al. Transcatheter aortic valve implantation in failed bioprosthetic surgical valves. JAMA 2014; 312:162–170.

15. Iung B, Nicoud-Houel A, Fondard O, et al. Temporal trends in percutaneous mitral commissurotomy over a 15-year period. Eur Heart J 2004; 25:701–707.

16. Bouleti C, Iung B, Laouénan C, et al. Late results of percutaneous mitral commissurotomy up to 20 years: development and validation of a risk score predicting late functional results from a series of 912 patients. Circulation 2012; 125:2119–2127.

17. McNeely CA, Vassileva CM. Long-term outcomes of mitral valve repair versus replacement for degenerative disease: a systematic review. Curr Cardiol Rev 2015; 11:157–162.

18. Chiam PTL, Ruiz CE. Percutaneous transcatheter mitral valve repair: a classification of the technology. JACC Cardiovasc Interv 2011; 4:1–13.

19. Fucci C, Sandrelli L, Pardini A, et al. Improved results with mitral valve repair using new surgical techniques. Eur J Cardiothorac Surg 1995; 9:621–626 discuss 626–627.

20. Alegria-Barrero E, Chan PH, Foin N, et al. Concept of the central clip: when to use one or two MitraClips®. EuroIntervention 2014; 9:1217–1224.

21. Feldman T, Kar S, Rinaldi M (for the EVEREST Investigators) et al. Percutaneous mitral repair with the MitraClip system: safety and midterm durability in the initial EVEREST (Endovascular Valve Edge-to-Edge REpair Study) cohort. J Am Coll Cardiol 2009; 54:686–694.

22. Mauri L, Foster E, Glower DD, et al. 4-year results of a randomized controlled trial of percutaneous repair versus surgery for mitral regurgitation. J Am Coll Cardiol 2013; 62:317–328.

23. Seiffert M, Conradi L, Baldus S, et al. Transcatheter mitral valve-in-valve implantation in patients with degenerated bioprostheses. JACC Cardiovasc Interv 2012; 5:341–349.

24. Wilbring M, Alexiou K, Tugtekin SM, et al. Pushing the limits-further evolutions of transcatheter valve procedures in the mitral position, including valve-in-valve, valve-in-ring, and valve-in-native-ring. J Thorac Cardiovasc Surg 2014; 147:210–219.

25. Meadows JJ, Moore PM, Berman DP, et al. Use and performance of the Melody Transcatheter Pulmonary Valve in native and postsurgical, nonconduit right ventricular outflow tracts. Circ Cardiovasc Interv 2014; 7:374–380.

26. Ribichini F, Pesarini G, Feola M, et al. Transcatheter tricuspid valve implantation by femoral approach in trivalvular heart disease. Am J Cardiol 2013; 112:1051–1053.

27. Lilly SM, Rome J, Anwaruddin S, et al. How should I treat prosthetic tricuspid stenosis in an extreme surgical risk patient? EuroIntervention 2013; 9:407–409.

28. Lauten A, Ferrari M, Hekmat K, et al. Heterotopic transcatheter tricuspid valve implantation: first-in-man application of a novel approach to tricuspid regurgitation. Eur Heart J 2011; 32:1207–1213.

29. Cullen MW, Cabalka AK, Alli OO, et al. Transvenous, antegrade Melody valve-in-valve implantation for bioprosthetic mitral and tricuspid valve dysfunction: a case series in children and adults. JACC Cardiovasc Interv 2013; 6:598–605.

Chapter 7

The elderly patient with aortic stenosis

Raj Chelliah, Philip MacCarthy

INTRODUCTION

It is becoming apparent that the prevalence of valvular heart disease is higher than previously thought and this presents a significant burden on health-care systems worldwide. Valvular heart disease becomes increasingly common in elderly patients, which is why degenerative disease (of both the aortic and mitral valves) has become by far the commonest aetiology [1] (**Figure 7.1**). An ageing population and more accessible treatment options in the transcatheter era have renewed interest in how we assess and treat elderly patients with significant valve disease and aortic stenosis (AS), with the novel intervention of transcatheter aortic valve implantation (TAVI), which has driven this process. It has long been known that symptomatic patients with AS require valvular intervention to alter the otherwise abysmal prognosis, but several studies [2] have shown that patients are often denied valve replacement (**Figure 7.2**). The reasons for this are not clear but assumptions about patients not being fit for surgical aortic valve replacement (sAVR), possibly made by physicians not qualified to make that decision, and lack of sophisticated assessment of the operative risk are clearly relevant. This was particularly the case before the TAVI era and Heart Teams around the world are in the process of unmasking and treating the hidden burden of AS that has been present for some time.

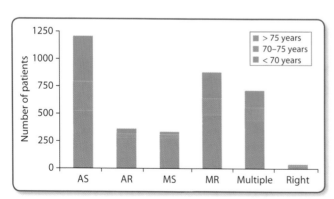

Figure 7.1 Age distribution according to the type of valvular heart disease in 3547 patients with native valve disease in the Euro Heart Survey. Aortic stenosis and mitral regurgitation are predominantly more common in the elderly patients. AR, aortic regurgitation; AS, aortic stenosis; MR, mitral regurgitation; MS, mitral stenosis; Multiple, multiple valve disease; Right, right sided heart disease.

Raj Chelliah MBChB MRCP, Department of Cardiology, King's College Hospital, London, UK

Philip MacCarthy BSc MBChB PhD FRCP, Department of Cardiology, King's College Hospital, Denmark Hill, London, UK. Email: philip.maccarthy@nhs.net (for correspondence)

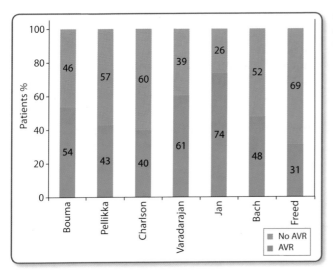

Figure 7.2 Composite of studies showing poor uptake and an unmet need for sAVR [36–42].

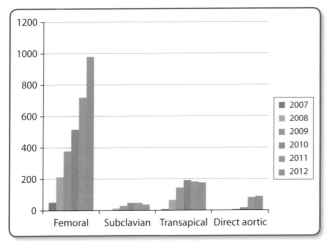

Figure 7.3 Transcatheter aortic valve implantation access route choice in the United Kingdom. This shows the expansion of the transfemoral route as the favoured choice of access, largely due to the lower complication rate.

Outcomes of sAVR remain excellent, but as our experience with TAVI expands, this minimally invasive approach gains appeal, particularly, for patients. Evolving technology and competent Heart Team assessment have made the procedure more predictable, with reducing rates of vascular injury, paravalvar aortic regurgitation and stroke. Smaller calibre delivery systems increase the number of patients eligible for a fully percutaneous procedure. This is reflected in the UK-TAVI data, which show increasing use of the transfemoral approach with consistently good outcomes (**Figure 7.3**) [3]. With this evolution have come shorter lengths of hospital stay and faster patient recovery times. It remains to be seen whether the current move towards performing these procedures under conscious sedation without a general anaesthetic will improve this further. Postprocedure delirium, pulmonary atelectasis and chest infection may be less common when general anaesthesia is avoided.

The classical teaching is that while AS remains asymptomatic, it is safe, and many patients remain under review with echocardiographic surveillance in clinics around the world. However, when symptoms occur everything changes and estimated survival at 2 years is only 50% [4]. Much of the data that supported this original assumption are outdated and were gathered from younger patients with less comorbidity suffering from rheumatic or bicuspid AS, rather than degenerative, calcific AS. Moreover, the point at which elderly patients (often with substantial comorbidity and limited mobility) become symptomatic is very often difficult to establish. The clinical reality is more difficult than the binary, classical teaching.

As transcatheter techniques become more mature; with decreasing complications, an established evidence base and strong data to suggest equivalence to sAVR, physicians may wish to offer earlier, less invasive valve intervention in certain patient subgroups (**Table 7.1**). This inevitably appeals to patients, who often mentioned the recovery time as an important factor in their preference for minimally invasive procedures to open surgery. Recent versions of both the European Society of Cardiology [5] and the American Heart association/American College of Cardiology (AHA/ACC) [6] guidelines have been published and there is a move to considering aortic valve 'intervention' rather than only sAVR in their advice. The guidelines also advocate obtaining further haemodynamic, symptomatic and anatomical data to assess valve disease severity in challenging cases.

VALVULAR ASSESSMENT AND ECHOCARDIOGRAPHIC SURVEILLANCE

The prognosis of truly asymptomatic patients with severe AS is relatively good, but there is no doubt that once the AS is severe enough to upset cardiac physiology and cause symptoms, the prognosis deteriorates rapidly (**Figure 7.4**) [7]. Valvular intervention has

Table 7.1 Characteristics of those who underwent valve intervention*						
	Aortic stenosis n = 512	Aortic regurgitation n = 119	Mitral stenosis n = 112	Mitral regurgitation n = 155	Multiple valve disease n = 185	Previous intervention n = 164
Age ≥ years (%)	54.3	19.3	17.9	31.6	25.4	33.5
Symptoms NYHA class (%)						
Class I	15.8	20.7	5.4	15.0	7.2	14.1
Class II	37.1	31.9	31.3	27.5	18.2	18.4
Class III	38.8	36.2	58.9	42.5	48.6	44.8
Class IV	8.3	11.2	4.4	15.0	26.0	22.7
Left ventricular ejection fraction (%)						
<30%	2.9	2.7	0	3.5	0.6	2.7
30–50%	16.4	21.8	8.7	16.2	21.6	15.4
50–60%	24.2	36.4	32.7	17.6	40.1	25.5
≥60%	56.5	39.1	58.6	62.7	37.7	56.4

Sixteen patients operated on for right-sided valve disease are not detailed.

*A large proportion of patients who undergo valvular intervention are symptomatic in New York Heart Association Class III–IV.

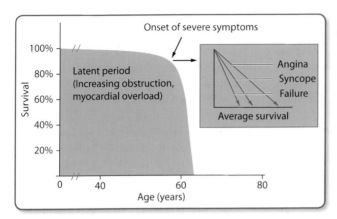

Figure 7.4 The natural history of aortic stenosis. At onset of symptoms, survival deteriorates rapidly.

therefore always been predicated upon the absence or presence of symptoms. In certain cohorts, however, the advent of symptoms may not necessarily be obvious. Elderly patients with reduced mobility and symptoms attributable to other comorbidities (e.g. airways disease, coronary artery disease, coexistent valve disease, frailty and immobility) may enhance the complexity of decision making. The Heart Team must, therefore, go beyond the mere presence or absence of symptoms when considering the risk–benefit ratio of aortic valve intervention.

Otto et al [8] concluded that even in asymptomatic patients, severe AS, defined by a jet velocity of 4 m/s or more, places the patients in a very poor prognostic category; 80% of patients with a jet velocity of 4 m/s eventually progress to symptoms requiring valve replacement. Conversely, only 35% of patients with a jet velocity of between 3 and 4 m/s progress to valve replacement over the same time period. This would signify that perhaps we should be intervening sooner than we currently are in the 'real world', and more widespread use of surveillance echocardiograms has possibly changed our practice in this regard. However, it has also become clear that we should not rely on one echo metric alone while assessing severity of AS. The jet velocity can sometimes be misleading, e.g. low-flow, low-gradient AS. In these cases, other echo features, such as left ventricular (LV) size/stroke volume and valve area, may play a vital role in contributing to the decision making. Rate of progress of AS, degree of calcification of the valve and severity of LV hypertrophy are also important – all metrics that can be observed and monitored during echocardiographic surveillance.

The role of the 'valve stress echo'

A 'valve stress echo' can assist exercise testing to assess exercise capacity, fall in blood pressure (BP) or ST-segment change, or malignant arrhythmias (ventricular tachycardia or conduction defects). The exercise can be performed on a treadmill or a static bicycle, the latter often being easier in elderly patients. Such a test can often simply establish whether the patient is truly asymptomatic on exercise – often symptoms become apparent early on that were not acknowledged in the history.

In a less-mobile patient, intravenous dobutamine stress is still a useful tool for further assessment of valve lesion severity [9–12]. The low-dose dobutamine stress echo can assess both the appropriate increase in valve area in response to increased transvalvular gradients and also contractile reserve in patients with LV dysfunction. In daily practice, valve stress echoes should be used in the following patient groups:

- Patients with an indeterminate severity of AS, e.g. low-gradient, low-flow AS (which may be due to poor LV function or may be paradoxical – caused by a small LV cavity and consequent small stroke volume)
- Patients with echocardiographically severe AS but no apparent symptoms
- Patients with known coronary disease to assess myocardial ischaemia
- Patients with severe depression of LV systolic function to assess contractile reserve – a key predictor of response to aortic valve intervention
- Patients with significant disease of other valves (e.g. mitral regurgitation) in addition to AS

Pharmacological testing is completely unable to reproduce the natural haemodynamic physiology during exercise. Conventional exercise testing, therefore, has advantages in obtaining objective evidence of exercise capacity, actual symptoms and BP response but does not allow for real-time Doppler assessment during incremental stages of exercise. The bicycle exercise stress echocardiogram may be helpful in that it allows more natural physiological changes during exercise and real-time Doppler assessment can be made at all the various stages of exercise and correspondent BP.

The current data indicate that an increase in the transaortic pressure gradient by >18 mmHg during exercise is an independent predictor of cardiac events during a follow-up period of 15 months [12]. Studies have corroborated this by assessing asymptomatic patients with moderate-to-severe AS with exercise stress echocardiography and established that an increase in exercise-induced mean gradient of >20 mmHg is a predictor of events and may provide additional prognostic information [13]. Heart Teams and valve clinics are increasingly using valve stress echo protocols, but widespread use of the investigation is affected by the relative lack of experience and technical ability to perform the test. Moreover, there is still a lack of data validating changes in valve stress echocardiographic parameters and their precise prognostic meaning.

CT calcium scoring of the aortic valve has also been used to predict outcomes in severe AS [14]. However, the data on this are less robust. Preliminary data do indicate that the degree of calcification may predict progression and development of symptoms. The 'calcium score' has also been shown to predict a worse long-term mortality in patients with low-flow, low-gradient severe AS [15]. There is no doubt that the degree and distribution of calcification of the aortic valve are now extremely important in assessing these patients, both in the surveillance phase and when deciding whether to intervene.

THE SPIRALLING ADVERSE EFFECTS OF AORTIC STENOSIS

The natural history and progression of AS present a complex interplay of adaptive responses, which initially aim to maintain normal haemodynamics and physiology, but eventually decompensate to cause rapid clinical deterioration. Timing the aortic valve intervention prior to this spiralling of adverse effects is key because the risks of intervention rise rapidly thereafter and patients should not have to become critically ill to 'earn' their definitive treatment. Many features of advancing calcific AS have adverse effects on the outcome of subsequent valve intervention and, clearly, as the risk of intervention decreases, the risk–benefit balance will favour earlier treatment. These disease features include increasing LV hypertrophy, diastolic dysfunction, subendocardial ischaemia, progression of valvular calcification, myocardial fibrosis and arrhythmias and eventually LV dilatation, functional mitral regurgitation, pulmonary hypertension and LV systolic decompensation and dysfunction.

Left ventricular hypertrophy and diastolic dysfunction

LV hypertrophy is itself an adverse prognostic indicator [16,17]. A number of different patterns of hypertrophy and adaptation have been described [18], and the degree of severity of AS does not correlate well with the degree of hypertrophy [19–21]. Careful characterisation of LV morphology/physiology helps the physicians to guide and predict outcomes and physiological changes perioperatively. The diastolic dysfunction may be multifactorial as a large proportion of patients may have hypertension, diabetes mellitus and atherosclerosis.

Subendocardial ischaemia

LV hypertrophy often results in subendocardial ischaemia, particularly at high heart rates. The subendocardium is at risk when ischaemia has high LV end diastolic pressures, particularly in the presence of coronary artery disease. Ischaemia increases not only the risk of sudden death but also the risk of any aortic valve intervention.

Calcification of the valve

The degree of calcification correlates with the degree of AS [22]. It has been found that it also predicts progression of AS, prognosis and the development of symptoms [23]. While some degree of calcification may be essential to ensure anchoring of a transcatheter valve, extensive and eccentric calcification increases the complexity of the procedure. Paravalvular leaks post-TAVI are more common in eccentrically and heavily calcified valves and paravalvular regurgitation is a known indicator of poor prognosis following TAVI [24]. Therefore, quantifying and timing intervention with the adequate amount of aortic valve calcification to ensure procedural success may be a focus in the future, prior to detrimental or eccentric calcification and increased procedural risk.

Failure of systolic contraction

LV systolic dysfunction is a strong predictor of adverse outcomes in aortic valve intervention [25]. This may represent the 'burnt-out' phase of the disease spectrum with subsequent LV dilatation and functional mitral regurgitation. There is evidence to suggest that myocardial fibrosis begins in the hypertrophic phase of the disease process [26,27]. However, we know that most patients with low-flow, low-gradient AS, but with contractile reserve, who undergo sAVR, demonstrate a significant improvement in LV ejection fraction and have a good long-term survival [28,29].

SAVR VERSUS TAVI: THE CURRENT EVIDENCE

The Placement of Aortic Transcatheter Valves (PARTNER) A [30] trial randomised high-risk patients according to the Society of Thoracic Surgeons (STS) score to either transcatheter or sAVR. The rate of death at 1 year from any cause was similar in both groups (24.2% vs. 26.8%; $P = 0.44$). However, complications differed in the two groups: there were higher rates of vascular injury (11.0% vs. 3.2%, $P < 0.001$ at 30 days) and stroke (5.1% vs. 2.4%; $P = 0.07$ at 1 year) in the transcatheter group but higher rates of major bleeding (19.5% vs. 9.3%; $P < 0.001$) and new onset atrial fibrillation (16.0% vs. 8.6%, $P = 0.06$) in the surgical group. The equivalence in mortality has now been shown to persist for at least 2 years.

The PARTNER B [31] trial randomised patients with severe AS who were not considered by the STS score to be suitable candidates for surgery. Standard 'medical therapy' (which included balloon valvuloplasty in 84%) was compared with TAVI. There was a dramatic 20% absolute improvement in survival at 1 year with TAVI, with the survival curve continuing to diverge at 1 year. The rate of death from any cause was 30.7% with transcatheter aortic valve replacement (AVR) versus 50.7% with standard therapy (hazard ratio with transcatheter replacement 0.55; $P < 0.001$). Longer-term persistence of benefit has been shown.

The recently published US Pivotal Trial [32] utilising the CoreValve selfexpanding valve is equally impressive. Mortality from any cause at 1 year in 795 randomised patients was significantly lower in the TAVI group than in the surgical group (14.2% vs. 19.1%), with an absolute reduction in the risk of 4.9% points (upper boundary of the 95% confidence interval, –0.4; $P < 0.001$ for noninferiority; $P = 0.04$ for superiority). TAVI was also noninferior with respect to echocardiographic indices of valve stenosis, functional status and quality of life.

It is, therefore, evident that both of the TAVI devices in commercial use demonstrate good outcomes which are sustained, shown so far out to several years. This has been shown in the inoperable (PARTNER B) as well as the high-risk (PARTNER A) patient cohorts. Data in the intermediate-risk group is currently being gathered (in the UK-TAVI, SURTAVI and PARTNER II Trials). Further clinical experience (both in the procedure and in case selection), technological development in device design and three-dimensional imaging and more sophisticated device sizing will all contribute to a further reduction in the risk of the procedure, making TAVI a very appealing and safe alternative to sAVR in certain patient populations.

PROCEDURAL RISK

The STS score and the EuroScore are currently the most widely used risk-scoring systems for the prediction of mortality postcardiac surgery. These scores were developed predominantly in low-to-intermediate risk cohorts of patients undergoing standard cardiac operations and do not accurately represent elderly patients undergoing sAVR or TAVI. Such scoring systems fail to take into account factors less easily quantifiable, such as patient frailty, mobility or psychological state/motivation. Moreover, they often exclude specific disease states which have direct impact on perioperative outcome, e.g. liver disease, 'porcelain aorta' or previous thoracic radiotherapy. The Heart Team therefore uses these scores only as a guide, and a more sophisticated, holistic assessment is needed to accurately tailor appropriate valve therapy.

Frailty may be challenging to assess appropriately, but the AHA/ACC guidelines suggest using a limited evaluation: no frailty (able to perform all activities of daily living and perform a 5-m walk in <6 s), mild degree of frailty (unable to perform one activity of daily living or unable to perform a 5-m walk in <6 s) and moderate-to-severe degree of frailty (unable to perform ≥2 activities of daily living). It is evident that more accurate and predictive risk scores are required, especially in selecting patients for transcatheter therapies. Procedural risk needs to be discussed with the patients so that an informed decision may be made. Involving the patient in the discussion is vital and the patient should be a key member of the Heart Team. Contemporary Heart Teams often invite patients to these clinical discussions and it has been shown that this often expedites clinical decisions [33].

EVOLUTION OF TAVI AND COST-EFFECTIVENESS

Transcatheter technology is evolving rapidly and, with the advent of newer devices, it is predicted that the periprocedural complications will fall and will eventually match the excellent outcomes with sAVR. There are a number of newer valve types emerging in the market. The Sapien 3 (Edwards Lifesciences, Irvine, CA, USA), Evolut R (Medtronic, Minneapolis, MN, USA), Lotus (Boston Scientific, MA, USA), Direct Flow (Direct Flow Medical, Santa Rosa, CA, USA) and the JenaValve (JenaValve Technology GmbH, Munich, Germany) have all progressed and been designed with specific technology aimed at reducing periprocedural complications. These include reducing paraprosthetic aortic regurgitation and reducing vascular complications and strokes with lower-profile delivery catheters. It remains to be seen whether outcome data support the aspirations of these devices.

Finally, it is conceivable that intervening early and at an appropriate stage of AS will be a more cost-effective strategy. The reality of the current system is that patients have to decompensate significantly to 'earn' their intervention. This often involves prolonged hospital admission (often with pulmonary oedema), with inhospital transfer to the local tertiary centre. Indeed, many patients eventually undergoing sAVR or TAVI have had several admissions with decompensation of their clinical state. Then they go on to have a higher-risk procedure, possibly with a longer length of postoperative hospital stay. An earlier, lower-risk procedure may be a more cost-effective approach. There have been studies showing that TAVI is likely to be cost-effective both in patients who are ineligible for sAVR [34] and in patients who are high risk [35].

Key points for clinical practice

- Optimal management of patients with AS is done with a functional, multidisciplinary Heart Team.
- The key to this management is appropriate case selection and the process of tailoring the optimal aortic valve intervention to the right patient.
- Timely intervention is vital to achieve the goal of satisfactory longer-term outcomes.
- This is a rapidly advancing field with constantly evolving technology in which we have to be careful to perform within the current evidence base.
- The TAVI procedure over the past 5 years has become safer and more predictable, especially via the transfemoral route, with recent major advances in the reduction in paravalvar AR and vascular complications.
- The traditional simplistic model of care of AS which divides patients according to the presence or absence of symptoms and allows the latter group to merely re-attend outpatient clinics for surveillance echocardiograms no longer applies in the modern era of valve disease management.

- Patients should be exposed to the Heart Team at an early stage and both clinical and echocardiographic assessment should be sophisticated and proactive, with judicious use of functional tests such as the valve stress echo.

- Current evidence does not support aortic valve intervention in the truly asymptomatic patient, but the current literature is evolving rapidly and clinicians will have to move at the same speed.

REFERENCES

1. Lung G, Baron B, Butchart EG, et al. A prospective survey of patients with valvular heart disease in Europe: The Euro Heart Survey on Valvular Heart Disease. Eur Heart J 2003; 24:1231–243.
2. Bouma BJ, van den Brink RBA, van der Meulen JHP, et al. To operate or not on elderly patients with aortic stenosis: the decision and its consequences. Heart 1999; 82:143–148.
3. Moat NE, Ludman P, de Belder MA, et al. Long-term outcomes after transcatheter aortic valve implantation in high risk patients with severe aortic stenosis: the UK TAVI registry. J Am Coll Cardiol 2011; 58:2130–2138.
4. Lester SJ, Heilbron B, Gin K, et al. The natural history and rate of progression of aortic stenosis. Chest 1998; 113:1109–1114.
5. Vahanian A, Alfieri O, Andreotti F, et al. Guidelines on the management of valvular heart disease (version 2012): the Joint Task Force on the management of valvular heart disease of the European Society of Cardiology (ESC) and the European Association of Cardio-Thoracic Surgery (EACTS); ESC Committee for Practice Guidelines (CPG); Joint Task Force on the Management of Valvular Heart Disease of the European Society of Cardiology (ESC); European Association for Cardio-Thoracic Surgery (EACTS). Eur J Cardiothorac Surg 2012; 42:S1–S44.
6. Nishimura RA, Otto CM, Bonow RO, et al. 2014 AHA/ACC guidelines for the management of patients with valvular heart disease: a report of the American College of Cardiology/American Heart Association Task Force on Practice Guidelines. J Am Coll Cardiol 2014; 63:2438–2488.
7. Ross J Jr, Braunwald E. Aortic stenosis. Circulation 1968; 38:61–67.
8. Otto CM, Burwash IG, Legget M, et al. Prospective study of asymptomatic valvular aortic stenosis. Clinical, echocardiographic, and exercise predictors of outcome. Circulation 1997; 95:2262–2270.
9. Lin SS, Roger VL, Pascoe R, et al. Dobutamine stress Doppler hemodynamics in patients with aortic stenosis: feasibility, safety, and surgical correlations. Am Heart J 1998; 136:1010–1016.
10. Monin JL, Monchi M, Gest V, et al. Aortic stenosis with severe left ventricular dysfunction and low transvalvular pressure gradients: risk stratification by low-dose dobutamine echocardiography. J Am Coll Cardiol 2001; 37:2101–2107.
11. Clavel MA, Fuchs C, Burwash IG, et al. Predictors of outcomes in low-flow, low-gradient aortic stenosis: results of the multicenter TOPAS Study. Circulation 2008; 118:S234–S242.
12. Lancellotti P, Lebois F, Simon M, et al. Prognostic importance of quantitative exercise Doppler echocardiography in asymptomatic valvular aortic stenosis. Circulation 2005; 112:I377–I382.
13. Maréchaux S, Hachicha Z, Bellouin A, et al. Usefulness of exercise stress echocardiography for risk stratification of true asymptomatic patients with aortic valve stenosis. Eur Heart J 2010; 31:1390–1397.
14. Cowell SJ, Newby DE, Burton J, et al. Aortic valve calcification on computed tomography predicts the severity of aortic stenosis. Clin Radiol 2003; 58:712–716.
15. Aksoy O, Cam A, Agarwal S, et al. Significance of aortic valve calcification in patients with low-gradient low-flow aortic stenosis. Clin Cardiol 2014; 37:26–31.
16. Pellikka PA, Sarano ME, Nishimura RA, et al. Outcome of 622 adults with asymptomatic, hemodynamically significant aortic stenosis during prolonged follow-up. Circulation 2005; 111:3290–3295.
17. Cioffi G, Faggiano P, Vizzardi E, et al. Prognostic effect of inappropriately high left ventricular mass in asymptomatic severe aortic stenosis. Heart 2011; 97:301–307.
18. Dweck MR, Boon NE, Newby DE. Calcific aortic stenosis: a disease of the valve and the myocardium. J Am Coll Cardiol 2012; 60:1854–1856.
19. Salcedo EE, Korzick DH, Currie PJ, et al. Determinants of left ventricular hypertrophy in patients with aortic stenosis. Cleve Clin J Med 1989; 56:590–596.

20. Kupari M, Turto H, Lommi J. Left ventricular hypertrophy in aortic valve stenosis: preventive or promotive of systolic dysfunction and heart failure? Eur Heart J 2005; 26:1790–1796.
21. Gunther S, Grossman W. Determinants of ventricular function in pressure-overload hypertrophy in man. Circulation 1979; 59:679–688.
22. Cowell SJ, Newby DE, Burton J, et al. Aortic valve calcification on computed tomography predicts the severity of aortic stenosis. Clin Radiol 2003; 58:712–716.
23. Rosenhek R, Binder T, Porenta G, et al. Predictors of outcome in severe, asymptomatic aortic stenosis. N Engl J Med 2000; 343:611–617.
24. Gotzmann M, Korten M, Bojara W, et al. Long-term outcome of patients with moderate and severe prosthetic aortic valve regurgitation after transcatheter aortic valve implantation. Am J Cardiol 2012; 110:1500–1506.
25. Lund O, Flo C, Jensen FT, et al. Left ventricular systolic and diastolic function in aortic stenosis. Prognostic value after valve replacement and underlying mechanisms. Eur Heart J 1997; 18:1977–1987.
26. Galiuto L, Lotrionte M, Crea F, et al. Impaired coronary and myocardial flow in severe aortic stenosis is associated with increased apoptosis: a transthoracic Doppler and myocardial contrast echocardiography study. Heart 2006; 92:208–212.
27. Anderson KR, Sutton MG, Lie JT. Histopathological types of cardiac fibrosis in myocardial disease. J Pathol 1979; 128:79–85.
28. Monin JL, Quere JP, Monchi M, et al. Low-gradient aortic stenosis: operative risk stratification and predictors for long-term outcome: a multicenter study using dobutamine stress hemodynamics. Circulation 2003; 108:319–324.
29. Quere JP, Monin JL, Levy F, et al. Influence of preoperative left ventricular contractile reserve on postoperative ejection fraction in low-gradient aortic stenosis. Circulation 2006; 113:1738–1744.
30. Elmariah S, Palacios IF, McAndrew T, et al. Outcomes of transcatheter and surgical aortic valve replacement in high-risk patients with aortic stenosis and left ventricular dysfunction: results from the Placement of Aortic Transcatheter Valves (PARTNER) trial (cohort A). Circ Cardiovasc Interv 2013; 6:604–614.
31. Leon MB, Smith CR, Mack M, et al. Transcatheter aortic-valve implantation for aortic stenosis in patients who cannot undergo surgery. N Engl J Med 2010; 363:1597–1607.
32. Reardon MJ, Adams DH, Coselli JS, et al. Self-expanding transcatheter aortic valve replacement using alternative access sites in symptomatic patients with severe aortic stenosis deemed extreme risk of surgery. J Thorac Cardiovasc Surg 2014; 148:2869–2876.
33. Showkathali R, Chelliah R, Brickham B, et al. Multi-disciplinary clinic: next step in 'Heart Team' approach for TAVI. Int J Cardiol 2014; 174:453–455.
34. Eaton J, Mealing S, Thompson J, et al. Is trancatheter aortic valve implantation (TAVI) a cost-effective treatment in patients who are ineligible for surgical aortic valve replacement? A systematic review of economic evaluations. J Med Econ 2014; 17:365–375.
35. Fairbairn TA, Meads DM, Hulme C, et al. The cost-effective of transcatheter aortic valve implantation versus surgical aortic valve replacement in patients with severe aortic stenosis at high operative risk. Heart 2013; 99:914–920.
36. Bouma BJ, Van Den Brink RB, Van Der Meulen JH, et al. To operate or not on elderly patients with aortic stenosis: the decision and its consequences. Heart 1999; 82:143–148.
37. Pellikka PA, Sarano ME, Nishimura RA, et al. Outcome of 622 adults with asymptomatic, hemodynamically significant aortic stenosis during prolonged follow-up. Circulation 2005; 111:3290–3295.
38. Charlson E, Legedza AT, Hamel MB. Decision-making and outcomes in severe symptomatic aortic stenosis. J Heart Valve Dis 2006; 15:312–321.
39. Varadarajan P, Kapoor N, Banscal RC, Pai RG. Clinical profile and natural history of 453 nonsurgically managed patients with severe aortic stenosis. Ann Thorac Surg 2006; 82:2111–2115.
40. Jan F, Andreev M, Mori N, Janosik B, Sagar K. Unoperated patients with severe symptomatic aortic stenosis. Circulation 2009; 120:S753.
41. Bach DS, Siao D, Girard SE, et al. Evaluation of patients with severe symptomatic aortic stenosis who do not undergo aortic valve replacement: the potential role of subjectively overestimated operative risk. Circ Cardiovasc Qual Outcomes 2009; 2:533–539.
42. Freed BH, Sugeng L, Furlong K, et al. Reasons for nonadherence to guidelines for aortic valve replacement in patients with severe aortic stenosis and potential solutions. Am J Cardiol 2010; 105:1339–1342.

Chapter 8

Heart failure with preserved ejection fraction

Grace Lin, Peter A Brady

INTRODUCTION

Heart failure as a clinical syndrome has been recognised for centuries. With the advent of cardiac imaging procedures to investigate better and to determine the pathophysiology of heart failure, recognition that heart failure was the result of reduced ventricular function was clearly established, and the development of targeted therapeutics for heart failure with reduced ejection fraction (EF) became possible. The notion that abnormal diastolic, as opposed to systolic dysfunction, could lead to a syndrome of congestion, and reduced cardiac reserve is more recent and less intuitive. However, it is now apparent that 'diastolic heart failure' or heart failure with preserved ejection fraction (HFpEF) accounts for approximately half of all patients with heart failure, with a prevalence ranging from 40% to 70% depending upon the definition of 'preserved' EF [1–4]. With advances in the understanding of the syndrome of HFpEF, the American College of Cardiology (ACC), American Heart Association (AHA) and European Society of Cardiology (ESC) guidelines have recommend HFpEF as the preferred terminology, and defined preserved ejection fraction as EF ≥50% [2,3]. Importantly, these guidelines reflect three concepts: (1) HFpEF is not caused by diastolic dysfunction alone, (2) diastolic heart failure is present in conditions other than HFpEF and (3) EF ≥50% is a preserved, rather than, 'normal' EF [3].

Whether heart failure with reduced ejection fraction (HFrEF) and HFpEF are two different diseases or opposite ends of one disease spectrum remains the subject of debate. The coexistence of systolic and diastolic dysfunction in both HFrEF and HFpEF argues for one continuous disease spectrum, but observations from heart failure registries and population studies report a bimodal distribution for EF, suggesting two distinct heart failure populations [1,5]. In addition, HFrEF and HFpEF have distinctly different risk profiles, demographics and response to pharmacologic therapies [1,6], which will be discussed in this chapter.

EPIDEMIOLOGY

Compared with HFrEF, the patient with HFpEF is older, more likely to be female and more likely to have atrial fibrillation but less likely to have had a prior myocardial infarction [1,7–9].

Grace Lin MD, Heart Failure Services, Mayo Clinic, Rochester, USA

Peter A Brady MD FRCP, ECG and Heart Rhythm Monitoring Laboratory, Mayo Clinic, Rochester, MN, USA. Email: lin.grace@mayo.edu (for correspondence)

Gender differences between HFrEF and HFpEF are quite striking with women almost twice as likely to develop HFpEF than men, a difference which, at least in part, may be driven by a comparative higher risk for HFrEF in men, owing to the greater incidence of prior myocardial infarction [8]. However, women develop more pronounced diastolic dysfunction, greater age-related increase of ventricular and vascular stiffness, and concentric ventricular remodelling in response to hypertension, which may also contribute to the higher risk of HFpEF [10]. Hypertension is highly prevalent and frequently a presenting feature in acute decompensated HFpEF [1,7,9], although a longitudinal analysis of the Framingham Heart Study comparing the risk profiles of HFrEF to HFpEF found that hypertension was a specific predictor of incident HFrEF rather than HFpEF, whereas higher body mass index, smoking and atrial fibrillation predicted the onset of HFpEF [8].

Noncardiovascular comorbidities, typical of ageing populations, may be more prevalent in HFpEF than HFrEF and contribute to higher rates of nonheart failure-related hospitalisations and mortality, with increasing risk of hospitalisations as the number of associated comorbidities increases [1,7-9,11]. Specific comorbidities common in HFpEF include obesity, renal failure, chronic lung disease, stroke, liver disease, cancer and anaemia, and result in differences in cardiac structure and mortality among HFpEF patients with individual or combinations of comorbidities [9,12,13]. Diastolic dysfunction is common in diabetic patients, who tend to be younger and more often male compared with other HFpEF patients, and have higher left ventricular (LV) filling pressures and stiffer vasculature [12,13]. In contrast, anaemic patients with HFpEF and those with renal dysfunction are older, more often female and have worse survival [12,13]. Obese patients with HFpEF have paradoxically lower mortality when compared with those with normal body mass index, possibly due to more preserved systolic and vascular function despite greater concentric remodelling [12,13].

PATHOPHYSIOLOGY

In contrast to HFrEF, where the mechanism of impaired cardiac output is more readily conceptualised due to decreased EF and LV enlargement, the pathophysiology of HFpEF is complex and less intuitive. Historically, HFpEF was considered to be purely due to diastolic dysfunction, but it is now understood to have additional and multifactorial pathophysiology [14-16]. Since HFpEF can result from any one or more of multiple mechanisms, it is now evident that HFpEF is a more heterogeneous syndrome than HFrEF, with distinct phenotypes that have different clinical presentations and outcomes, and variations in cardiac structural remodelling (**Figure 8.1**) [13,17,18].

Diastolic dysfunction is caused by increased myocardial stiffness as a result of multiple factors including changes in cardiomyocyte stiffness as well as in collagen deposition and crosslinking in the extracellular matrix [15]. These changes lead to abnormal LV relaxation and increased LV filling pressures, and in HFpEF results in limited augmentation of stroke volume with exercise and during tachycardia simulated by atrial pacing [15,19,20]. Myocardial stiffness increases with senescence perhaps accounting for the predominance of HFpEF in elderly patients, although both HFpEF and asymptomatic diastolic dysfunction can occur in patients as young as 40-50 years old [4,15,19,21]. Asymptomatic diastolic dysfunction is present in up to 24% of community population cohorts, and of these, individuals with moderate-severe diastolic dysfunction and normal EF comprise a smaller subset (5.6%) [4,21]. However, only one in four individuals with asymptomatic diastolic

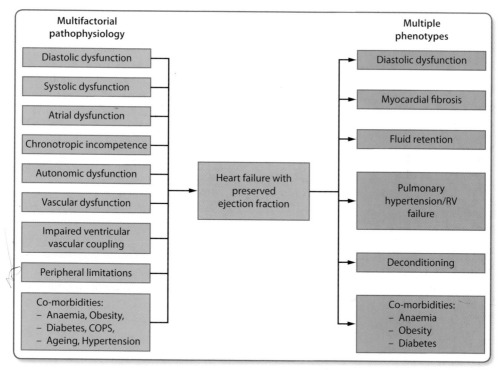

Figure 8.1 Multifactorial pathophysiology of heart failure with preserved ejection fraction (HFpEF). Multiple mechanisms contribute to the onset of HFpEF which result in distinct clinical phenotypes.

dysfunction eventually progressed to heart failure, underscoring the contribution of other mechanisms and comorbidities in the pathophysiology of HFpEF [4,21].

Despite preservation of EF, systolic function is also impaired in HFpEF [15,18]. Earlier studies observed decreased myocardial contractility in HFpEF compared with healthy and hypertensive controls with normal EF, as well as regional changes in systolic function detected by tissue Doppler techniques with echocardiography [15]. More recently, myocardial strain, a measurement of myocardial deformation and mechanics which permits assessment of longitudinal, radial and circumferential systolic function, has been utilised to characterise global systolic function in HFpEF in the Prospective Comparison of Angiotensin Receptor Neprilysin Inhibitor with Angiotensin Receptor Blocker (ARB) in Management of Heart Failure with Normal Ejection Fraction (PARAMOUNT) trial [18]. Compared with healthy and hypertensive controls with normal EF, longitudinal systolic strain is impaired in two-thirds of patients with HFpEF and circumferential systolic strain impaired in 40%, supporting the concept that systolic dysfunction is common in HFpEF [18].

Additional mechanisms that contribute to HFpEF are increased vascular stiffness, abnormal ventricular–vascular coupling, chronotropic incompetence, autonomic dysfunction, impaired peripheral vasodilation and skeletal muscle dysfunction [15]. A final common pathway could be systemic inflammation induced by the many comorbidities common in HFpEF leading to coronary vascular endothelial inflammation, myocardial remodelling and, eventually, heart failure [14].

The end result of this multifactorial pathophysiology is decreased cardiovascular reserve, dyspnoea and activity intolerance that is typical of HFpEF (**Table 8.1**). Dyspnoea during exertion reflects limited augmentation of cardiac output and heart rate during exercise. Systemic blood pressure is often labile in response to small fluctuations in volume or afterload. Pulmonary hypertension due to chronically elevated left-sided pressures and increased pulmonary vascular resistance is also common and increased during exercise, and eventually results in right ventricular dysfunction and increased mortality [22].

MORTALITY AND OUTCOMES

The hospital and short-term mortality of HFpEF is high but lower than in HFrEF [1,7]. Both the Organized Program to Initiate Lifesaving Treatment in Hospitalized Patients and the Acute Decompensated Heart Failure National Registries (ADHERE) demonstrated lower inhospital mortality in HFpEF compared with HFrEF patients (ADHERE: 2.9% vs. 3.9%, $P < 0.001$) [1,7]. Length of hospital stay, postdischarge 60–90-day mortality and rates of readmission were, however, similar [1,7]. HFpEF patients were equally likely to be discharged with persistent congestion, but fewer HFpEF patients required intensive care unit level care compared to HFrEF [1,7]. During the past two decades, the prevalence of HFpEF-related hospital admissions has continued to increase in contrast to HFrEF admissions, which have been relatively stable [11,23]. While the duration of hospitalisation for HFpEF and inhospital mortality has improved, postdischarge mortality and readmissions, mostly for noncardiovascular comorbidities, have increased [23–25].

Long-term survival of HFpEF patients is also poor and approaches that of HFrEF. A large community population study reported 1-year mortality of 29% and 5-year mortality of 65% in HFpEF, with similar rates in HFrEF, although the adjusted hazard ratio (HR) for death favoured HFpEF (HR 0.96, CI 0.92–1.00, $P < 0.01$) [11]. A large meta-analysis of >40,000 patients with heart failure observed a 32% lower risk of death over 3 years in HFpEF compared with HFrEF, but this difference was most significant for younger patients, <55 years old, and was less prominent in older adults, especially women >75 years old [26]. In the 'Get with the Guidelines' database of Medicare patients older than 65 years there was no significant difference in survival of HFpEF compared to HFrEF after risk adjustment (35.6 vs. 37.5% 1-year survival) [23].

Table 8.1 Changes in physiologic response to exercise with heart failure with preserved ejection fraction*		
Parameter	Normal	HFpEF
Heart rate	↑	Blunted response
Systolic blood pressure	↑	↑↑↑
Pulmonary capillary wedge pressure	↑ Slightly	↑↑↑
Peripheral vasodilation	↑	Impaired
Contractility	↑	Blunted response
Peripheral muscle oxygen extraction	↑	Impaired
Cardiac output	↑	Blunted response

*Augmentation of cardiac output, heart rate and peripheral vasodilation during exercise is blunted.
HFpEF, heart failure with preserved ejection fraction.

A diagnosis of HFpEF also does not protect against a subsequent decline in EF, a change that probably further impacts on long-term survival [5]. A community-based study observed that EF in HFpEF declines by as much as 6% per year over 5 years, with more prominent decline in older patients and those with coronary artery disease [5]. Each 5% decline in EF was associated with a 7% increase in mortality [5]. In HFrEF, use of evidence-based medical therapy can result in improvement in EF which may translate into improved survival. However, medical therapy does not provide a protective benefit against declining EF in HFpEF. Whether the trend for decreasing EF in some patients with HFpEF simply reflects the natural history or is the result of a subsequent specific injury or insult, such as ischaemia, is unclear [5].

DIAGNOSIS OF HFPEF

Whereas HFrEF can be diagnosed by imaging studies demonstrating decreased EF, the cardiac structural abnormalities that can be found in HFpEF are neither uniform nor unique to HFpEF. Concentric LV remodelling and hypertrophy, impaired ventricular strain and cardiac fibrosis are present in many but not all HFpEF patients; similarly, these structural abnormalities can be observed in other conditions [15,17,18]. HFpEF must also be distinguished from asymptomatic diastolic dysfunction and unexplained dyspnoea due to other causes. Diagnosis of HFpEF, therefore, requires simultaneous presence of clinical heart failure, diastolic dysfunction with increased LV filling pressures and normal EF [3,15,27]. One algorithm proposed by the Heart Failure and Echocardiography Associations of the ESC stipulates an LV end-diastolic pressure (LVEDP) >16 mmHg, pulmonary capillary wedge pressure (PCWP) >12 mmHg or E/e' ratio >8 (an echocardiographic estimate of PCWP) [27]. Although elevated natriuretic peptide levels [NT (N-terminal) pro-BNP (brain natriuretic peptide) > 220 pg/mL; BNP > 200 pg/mL] can supplement the diagnostic workup, because of the low sensitivity of the selected cut-off values in the ESC algorithm, they are not sufficient as independent criteria and evidence of increased LV filling pressures is still required [27]. Natriuretic peptide levels may be of more benefit to exclude HFpEF in a dyspnoeic patient without clear signs and symptoms of volume overload; an NT pro-BNP level of <120 pg/mL and BNP of <100 pg/mL have high negative predictive values to exclude HFpEF in this clinical scenario [27].

HFpEF can be readily diagnosed on the basis of the ESC criteria if congestion and elevated filling pressures are present at rest but these findings may be absent in early stage or well-compensated HFpEF [15]. In these patients, cardiac catheterisation or Doppler echocardiography to document increased filling pressures during exercise may be required to diagnose HFpEF. Guidelines for exercise haemodynamics in the diagnosis of HFpEF patients are less well defined than for resting haemodynamics. Since peak of PCWP is usually <20–33 mmHg or LVEDP <25 mmHg with exercise in healthy individuals, some studies have defined a pathologic response to diagnose HFpEF as PCWP or LVEDP >25 mmHg and mean pulmonary artery pressure >30 mmHg with exercise [28]. E/e' ratio (to estimate PCWP by echocardiography) is expected to remain stable throughout exercise in normal individuals; a rise in E/e' or right ventricular systolic pressure suggests a diagnosis of HFpEF by exercise stress echocardiography [29]. Although dobutamine can be utilised to increase heart rate during stress echocardiography it is less useful for diagnosis of HFpEF due to the direct haemodynamic effects of dobutamine that may cause a drop in diastolic pressure [29].

TREATMENT

In recognition of the importance of the clinical syndrome of heart failure, the ACC/AHA heart failure guidelines have focussed on its progressive nature and emphasised early recognition to enable earlier risk factor modification directed towards prevention or slowing of disease progression [7]. Specifically, four stages of heart failure are characterised: stage A, to include individuals at risk of heart failure developing but without evidence of structural heart disease or heart failure; stage B, individuals with evidence of structural heart disease but without overt heart failure; stage C, individuals with symptomatic heart failure; and stage D, patients with advanced heart failure [3]. Management of stage A patients is directed towards risk factor modification in both HFrEF and HFpEF. However, while medical therapies for stage B–D HFrEF are well established, disease-modifying therapies in stage B–D HFpEF are lacking (**Table 8.2**) [13,15,16,30].

Both angiotensin converting enzyme (ACE) inhibitors and ARBs are effective treatments for hypertension but have a neutral effect on mortality in HFpEF [3,15]. The perindopril in elderly people with chronic heart failure (PEP-CHF) study, a randomised trial that compared perindopril 4 mg daily to placebo, found no improvement in mortality or frequency of hospitalisations in the treatment group [15,30]. Similarly, the Candesartan in Heart Failure: Assessment of Mortality and Morbidity (CHARM-Preserved) trial randomised 3023 patients with heart failure and EF >40% to candesartan or placebo and did not demonstrate an impact on mortality; although fewer heart failure hospitalisations were observed in the group treated with candesartan [13,15,30]. The Irbesartan in Heart Failure with Preserved Systolic Function (I-PRESERVE) trial is the largest study of HFpEF patients to date; enrolling over 4000 patients either recently hospitalised or with advanced heart failure and randomised to irbesartan or placebo. The study observed no differences in mortality or decreases in subsequent cardiovascular hospitalisations with irbesartan [13,15,30].

Two drug classes, mineralocorticoid receptor antagonists (MRAs) and phosphodiesterase 5 (PDE5) inhibitors, improved diastolic dysfunction in HFpEF studies, but this effect has not translated into mortality benefit or improved functional capacity. Aldosterone mediates the progression of myocardial stiffness through multiple mechanisms, and indeed, small studies have demonstrated improvement in diastolic function parameters with aldosterone blockade using MRAs [13]. However, two randomised trials, the Aldosterone Receptor Blockade in Diastolic Heart Failure (Aldo-DHF) and the Treatment of Preserved Cardiac Function Heart Failure with an Aldosterone Antagonist (TOPCAT) investigated the use of spironolactone in HFpEF and found no improvement in exercise capacity, mortality, risk of sudden death or frequency of heart failure hospitalisations [13]. PDE5 inhibitors, such as sildenafil, modulate the nitric oxide (NO)–cyclic guanosine monophosphate (cGMP)–protein kinase G (PKG) pathway, which increases cardiomyocyte stiffness through alterations in myocyte architecture [13]. Although sildenafil reduced LV wall thickness and improved diastolic filling parameters in a small study of patients with HFpEF and pulmonary hypertension, the larger PDE5 Inhibition to Improve to Improve Clinical Status and Exercise Capacity in Heart failure with Preserved Ejection Fraction (RELAX) was unable to demonstrate improvements in peak oxygen consumption or 6-minute walk time after 24 weeks of treatment with sildenafil compared to placebo [13,15].

The few studies of beta-blockers and digoxin in HFpEF and have also shown a neutral effect on mortality although the frequency of hospitalisations decreased [2,30]. Both the

Table 8.2 Clinical trials of pharmacotherapy for heart failure with preserved ejection fraction

Trial	Year	Drug	No. of patients (no. assigned)	Ejection fraction	Inclusion criteria	Primary end point	Outcome
CHARM-Preserved [32]	2003	Angiotensin receptor blocker: Candesartan 32 mg daily vs. placebo	3023 1514 assigned to Candesartan	≥40%	Age >18 years NYHA II–IV Previous CV hospitalisation	CV death or HF hospitalisation	No difference in primary end point: 22% candesartan vs. 24% placebo (HR 0.89 95% CI 0.77–1.03, P = 0.118) Trend towards benefit on hospital admissions, no impact on CV mortality
SENIORS [33]	2005	Beta blocker: Nebivolol 10 mg daily vs. placebo	2128 1067 assigned to nebivolol	≥ 35% (36% of no. enrolled in study)	Age ≥ 70 years old Heart failure (HF) hospitalisation within 12 months	All-cause mortality or CV hospitalisation	Decrease in primary point: 31% nebivolol vs. 35% placebo (HR 0.86 95% CI 0.74–0.99, P = 0.039) Did not impact all-cause mortality No difference in outcome based on EF
Ancillary DIG Trial [34]	2006	Digoxin vs. placebo: Dose based on age, sex, weight, serum creatinine levels	988 492 assigned to digoxin	>45%	Normal sinus rhythm	HF hospitalisation or mortality	No difference in primary end point: 21% in digoxin vs. 24% placebo (HR 0.82, 95% CI 0.63–1.07, P = 0.136) Decrease in HF hospitalisations: 12% digoxin vs. 17% placebo in first 2 years (HR 0.66, 95% CI 0.73–1.36, P = 0.012)
PEP-CHF [35]	2006	ACE inhibitor: Perindopril 5 mg daily vs. placebo	850 424 assigned to perindopril	>40%	Age ≥ 70 years HF with hospitalisation within 6 months 3 of 9 clinical criteria for HF 2 of 4 echocardiographic criteria: increased LV wall thickness, diastolic dysfunction, LA enlargement, wall motion index 1.4–1.6	All-cause mortality or HF hospitalisation	No difference in primary end point: 24% perindopril vs. 25% placebo (HR 0.92, 95% CI 0.70–1.21, P = 0.545)

Table 8.2 continued...

I-PRESERVE [36]	2008	Angiotensin receptor blocker: Irbesartan 300 mg daily vs. placebo	4128 2067 assigned to irbesartan	≥45%	Age ≥ 60 years HF with hospitalisation within 6 months NYHA II–IV	All-cause mortality or CV hospitalisation	No difference in primary outcome: 36% irbesartan vs. 37% placebo (HR 0.95, 95% CI 0.86–1.05, P = 0.35)
PARAMOUNT [37]	2012	Angiotensin receptor neprilysin inhibitor: LCZ696 200 mg twice daily vs. valsartan 160 mg twice daily	308 149 assigned to LCZ696	≥45%	Age ≥ 40 years HF symptoms requiring diuretics SBP < 140 mmHg or < 160 mmHg on ≥ 3 antihypertensive drugs NT pro-BNP > 400 pg/mL GFR ≥ 30 cm³/min/1.73 m²	Change in baseline NT pro-BNP	Greater reduction in NT pro-BNP with LCZ696 compared to valsartan
Aldo-DHF7	2013	Mineralocorticoid receptor antagonist Spironolactone 25 mg daily vs. placebo	422 213 assigned to spironolactone	≥50%	Age ≥ 50 years NYHA II–III Diastolic dysfunction by echocardiography or atrial fibrillation at presentation Peak VO2 ≤ 25 mL/kg/ min	Change in diastolic function (E/e' ratio) and peak VO2 at 12 months	Decreased E/e' with spironolactone compared with placebo No difference in peak VO2 change with spironolactone compared to placebo
Aldo-DHF [38]	2013	Mineralocorticoid receptor antagonist: Spironolactone 25 mg daily vs. placebo	422 213 assigned to spironolactone	≥50%	Age ≥ 50 years NYHA II–III Diastolic dysfunction by echocardiography or AF at presentation Peak VO₂ ≤ 25 mL/kg/ min	Change in diastolic function (E/e' ratio) and peak VO₂ at 12 months	Decreased E/e' with spironolactone compared with placebo No difference in peak VO₂ change with spironolactone compared to placebo

Table 8.2 continued...

RELAXF [39]	2013	Phosphodiesterase 5 inhibitor: Sildenafil 20 mg three times daily vs. placebo	216 113 assigned to placebo	≥50%	NYHA II–IV Previous HF hospitalisation, requiring IV or chronic oral diuretics, ↑PCWP or LVEDP) Peak VO$_2$ ≤60% of predicted NT pro-BNP ≥ 400 pg/mL	Change in peak VO$_2$ at 24 weeks	No difference in peak VO$_2$ change with sildenafil compared to placebo
TOPCAT [40]w	2014	Mineralocorticoid receptor antagonist: Spironlactone 45 mg daily vs. placebo	3445 1722 assigned to spironolactone	≥ 45%	Age ≥ 50 years HF symptoms with hospitalisation within 12 months or BNP ≥ 100 pg/mL or NT pro-BNP ≥ 360 pg/mL SBP <140 mmHg or <160 mmHg on ≥3 antihypertensive drugs Serum K < 5.0 mmol/L	CV death, aborted cardiac arrest, or HF hospitalisation	No difference in primary end point: 18.6% spironolactone vs. 20.4% placebo (HR 0.89, 95% CI 0.77–1.04, P = 0.14)

ACE, angiotensin converting enzyme; Aldo-DHF, Aldosterone Receptor Blockade in Diastolic Heart Failure; CHARM, Candesartan in Heart Failure: Assessment of Mortality and Morbidity; CI, confidence interval; CV, cardiovascular; DIG, Digitalis Investigators Group; EF, Ejection fraction; GFR, glomerular filtration rate; HR, Hazard ratio, I-PRESERVE, irbesartan in heart failure with preserved systolic function; LA, Left atrial; LVEDP, Left ventricular end-diastolic pressure; NYHA, New York Heart Association; PCWP, pulmonary capillary wedge pressure; PEP-CHF, perindopril in elderly people with chronic heart failure; SBP, systolic blood pressure; SENIORS, Study of Effects of Nebivolol Intervention on Outcomes and Rehospitalisation in Seniors; TOPCAT, Treatment of Preserved Cardiac Function Heart Failure with an Aldosterone Antagonist.

Digitalis Investigators Group (DIG) and the Study of Effects of Nebivolol Intervention on Outcomes and Rehospitalisation in Seniors (SENIORS) included patients with variable definitions of 'preserved' EF (SENIORS: EF >35%; DIG ancillary trial: EF >45%. Overall SENIORS demonstrated a 14% reduction in the composite primary outcome of all mortality cause and cardiovascular hospitalisation with nebivolol independent of EF, but did not show a decrease in mortality alone [2,30]. The findings from DIG ancillary trial were similar to the DIG main trial with EF <45%; there was no impact on mortality but the use of digoxin decreased the need for heart failure hospitalisations [2].

Owing to the lack of evidence to support mortality or morbidity benefit of ACE inhibitors, ARBs, MRAs, PDE 5 inhibitors, beta-blockers or digoxin in HFpEF, neither the ACC/AHA nor ESC heart failure guidelines recommend the routine use of these drugs specifically for the treatment of HFpEF, although some drug classes may be indicated for treatment of risk factors [2,3]. In the absence of therapies which have an impact on mortality, the current management of HFpEF is directed towards prevention through risk factor modification, and symptom management. Diuretics and dietary modification of sodium and fluid intake are recommended to treat congestion. Exercise training has been shown to improve peak oxygen consumption and quality of life in HFpEF, and could improve symptoms related to activity intolerance and dyspnoea with exertion [13]. Beta-blockers are generally not indicated in HFpEF due to chronotropic incompetence but may be required for rate control of atrial fibrillation [2, 3].

The failure of clinical trials to demonstrate mortality benefit in HFpEF has been attributed to variable trial selection criteria resulting in recruitment of study cohorts without uniform disease pathophysiology or cardiac structure, but may also be due to the heterogeneous nature of HFpEF itself [13,30]. Future clinical trials and HFpEF treatment strategies may require targeting of specific therapies, to patients with a particular phenotype, rather than the more uniform approach to medical therapy that has been successful in HFrEF. For example, PDE5 inhibition may be beneficial only if pulmonary hypertension is present, and may be less advantageous in other HFpEF phenotypes [13]. The TOPCAT trial also found a significant interaction between treatment effect and patient recruitment strategy supporting the idea of targeted therapy to subgroups of HFpEF patients with similar pathophysiology and phenotype [13].

There are several ongoing and planned trials of HFpEF. The phase II PARAMOUNT trial compared the ARNI (Angiotensin Receptor-Neprilysin Inhibitor) LCZ696 to valsartan; ARNIs are expected to increase the bioavailability of natriuretic and vasodilator peptides [13]. PARAMOUNT demonstrated a greater change in measured serum NT pro-BNP and decrease in left atrial size with LCZ696 compared with valsartan but whether these effects on NT pro-BNP will translate into clinical benefit is being explored in the Efficacy and Safety of LCZ696 Compared to Valsartan, on Morbidity and Mortality in HFpEF (PARAGON-HF) trial [13]. Soluble guanylate cyclase stimulators such as riociguat target the NO–cGMP–PG pathway to increase NO-induced pulmonary vasodilation and may benefit patients with pulmonary hypertension [13]. Ivabradine, a selective I_f channel inhibitor, has been shown to reduce ventricular stiffness in an animal model, and short-term treatment has been associated with improved exercise tolerance in patients with high resting heart rates [13].

DEVICE THERAPY AND ARRHYTHMIAS

Implantable cardioverter defibrillator (ICD) and cardiac resynchronisation therapy (CRT) have proven survival and symptom benefit in patients with HFrEF but indications in HFpEF are less well defined. Left bundle branch block, a marker of electrical dyssynchrony as well as risk of sudden cardiac death in HFrEF, is less common in HFpEF and the clinical implication of mechanical dyssynchrony in HFpEF, especially in the absence of left bundle branch block, is controversial [31]. Sudden death risk in HFpEF is poorly understood compared with the situation in HFrEF, although the incidence of sudden death in HFpEF may be lower relative to death from progressive pump failure. EF has been central to risk stratification in HFrEF [31]. These same criteria cannot be applied to HFpEF and there is accumulating evidence that risk stratification beyond EF is needed even in HFrEF [31]. Biomarkers and ECG-derived criteria are potential risk markers in HFpEF but have not yet been adequately characterised [31]. In the light of these limited data, at present, the ACC, AHA and ESC guidelines do not recommend routine use of ICD for primary prophylaxis of sudden death, or CRT for treatment of symptomatic heart failure, in HFpEF [2,3]. Atrial pacing support with rate responsiveness may be of value in some patients with chronotropic incompetence but has yet to be proven in clinical trials [13]. While prevention and adequate rate control of atrial fibrillation may impact symptoms in HFpEF the benefit of advanced therapies such as left atrial ablation, at least on survival, is unclear.

CONCLUSION

HFpEF is heterogeneous clinical syndrome seemingly distinct from HFrEF. Therapies known to be proven in terms of symptoms and mortality benefit, have failed to show similar benefit in patients with HFpEF. Better understanding of the underlying mechanisms and pathophysiology of HFpEF can guide development of more effective therapeutic targets for prevention, symptom control and mortality benefit.

> **Key points for clinical practice**
>
> - HFpEF is a heterogeneous clinical syndrome with multifactorial pathophysiology accounting for half of patients with heart failure.
> - Ageing, female gender, hypertension, obesity and atrial fibrillation are commonly associated with HFpEF.
> - Physiologic response to exercise in HFpEF is altered, resulting in activity limitation.
> - HFpEF must be distinguished from asymptomatic diastolic dysfunction and dyspnoea due to other causes.
> - Long-term mortality in HFpEF is high.
> - No single pharmacologic therapy has been demonstrated to have mortality benefit in HFpEF.

REFERENCES

1. Fonarow GC, Stough WG, Abraham WT, et al. Characteristics, treatments, and outcomes of patients with preserved systolic function hospitalized for heart failure: a report from the OPTIMIZE-HF Registry. J Am Coll Cardiol 2007; 50:768–777.
2. McMurray JJV, Adamopoulos S, Anker SD, et al. ESC Guidelines for the diagnosis and treatment of acute and chronic heart failure 2012. Eur J Heart Fail 2012; 14:803–869.
3. Yancy CW, Jessup M, Bozkurt B, et al. 2013 ACCF/AHA guideline for the management of heart failure: a report of the American College of Cardiology Foundation/American Heart Association Task Force on Practice Guidelines. J Am Coll Cardiol 2013; 62:e147–e239.

4. Redfield MM, Jacobsen SJ, Burnett JC Jr, et al. Burden of systolic and diastolic ventricular dysfunction in the community: appreciating the scope of the heart failure epidemic. JAMA 2003; 289:194–202.
5. Dunlay SM, Roger VL, Weston SA, Jiang R, Redfield MM. Longitudinal changes in ejection fraction in heart failure patients with preserved and reduced ejection fraction. Circ Heart Fail 2012; 5:720–726.
6. Borlaug BA, Redfield MM, Diastolic and systolic heart failure are distinct phenotypes within the heart failure spectrum. Circulation 2011; 123:2006–2014.
7. Yancy CW, Lopatin M, Stevenson LW, De Marco T, Fonarow GC. Clinical presentation, management, and in-hospital outcomes of patients admitted with acute decompensated heart failure with preserved systolic function: a report from the cute Decompensated Heart Failure National Registry (ADHERE) Database. J Am Coll Cardiol 2006; 47:76–84.
8. Ho JE, Lyass A, Lee DS, et al. Predictors of new-onset heart failure: differences in preserved versus reduced ejection fraction. Circ Heart Fail 2013; 6:279–286.
9. Ather S, Chan W, Bozkurt B, et al. Impact of noncardiac comorbidities on morbidity and mortality in a predominantly male population with heart failure and preserved versus reduced ejection fraction. J Am Coll Cardiol 2012; 59:998–1005.
10. Gori M, Lam CSP, Gupta DK, et al. Sex-specific cardiovascular structure and function in heart failure with preserved ejection fraction. Eur J Heart Fail 2014; 16:535–542.
11. Owan TE, Hodge DO, Herges RM, et al. Trends in prevalence and outcome of heart failure with preserved ejection fraction. N Engl J Med 2006; 355:251–259.
12. Mohammed SF, Borlaug BA, Roger VL, et al. Comorbidity and ventricular and vascular structure and function in heart failure with preserved ejection fraction: a community-based study. Circ Heart Fail 2012; 5:710–719.
13. Senni M, Paulus WJ, Gavazzi A, et al. New strategies for heart failure with preserved ejection fraction: the importance of targeted therapies for heart failure phenotypes. Eur Heart J 2014; 35:2797–2815.
14. Paulus WJ, Tschöpe C. A novel paradigm for heart failure with preserved ejection fraction: comorbidities drive myocardial dysfunction and remodeling through coronary microvascular endothelial inflammation. J Am Coll Cardiol 2013; 62:263–271.
15. Borlaug BA, Paulus WJ. Heart failure with preserved ejection fraction: pathophysiology, diagnosis, and treatment. Eur Heart J 2011; 32:670–679.
16. Maeder MT, Kaye DM. Heart failure with normal left ventricular ejection fraction. J Am Coll Cardiol 2009; 53:905–918.
17. Kitzman DW, Upadhya B. Heart failure with preserved ejection fraction: a heterogenous disorder with multifactorial pathophysiology. J Am Coll Cardiol 2014; 63:457–459.
18. Kraigher-Krainer E, Shah AM, Gupta DK, et al. Impaired systolic function by strain imaging in heart failure with preserved ejection fraction. J Am Coll Cardiol 2014; 63:447–456.
19. Westermann D, Kasner M, Steendijk P, et al. Role of left ventricular stiffness in heart failure with normal ejection fraction. Circulation 2008; 117:2051–2060.
20. Zile MR, Baicu CF, Gaasch WH. Diastolic heart failure – abnormalities in active relaxation and passive stiffness of the left ventricle. N Engl J Med 2004; 350:1953–1959.
21. Kane GC, Karon BL, Mahoney DW, et al. Progression of left ventricular diastolic dysfunction and risk of heart failure. JAMA 2011; 306:856–863.
22. Borlaug BA. The pathophysiology of heart failure with preserved ejection fraction. Nat Rev Cardiol 2014; 11:507–515.
23. Cheng RK, Cox M, Neely ML, et al. Outcomes in patients with heart failure with preserved, borderline, and reduced ejection fraction in the Medicare population. Am Heart J 2014; 168:721–730.
24. Bueno H, Ross JS, Wang Y, et al. Trends in length of stay and short-term outcomes among Medicare patients hospitalized for heart failure: 1993–2008. JAMA 2010; 303:2141–2147.
25. Steinberg BA, Zhao X, Heidenreich PA, et al. Trends in patients hospitalized with heart failure and preserved left ventricular ejection fraction: prevalence, therapies, and outcomes. Circulation 2012; 126:65–75.
26. Meta Analysis Global Group in Chronic Heart Failure, The survival of patients with heart failure with preserved or reduced left ventricular ejection fraction: an individual patient data meta-analysis. Eur Heart J 2012; 33:1750–1757.
27. Paulus WJ, Tschöpe C, Sanderson JE, et al. How to diagnose diastolic heart failure: a consensus statement on the diagnosis of heart failure with normal left ventricular ejection fraction by the Heart Failure and Echocardiography Associations of the European Society of Cardiology. Eur Heart J 2007; 28:2539–2550.
28. Borlaug BA, Nishimura RA, Sorajja P, Lam CSP, Redfield MM. Exercise hemodynamics enhance diagnosis of early heart failure with preserved ejection fraction. Circ Heart Fail 2010; 3:588–595.

29. Oh JK, Kane GC. Diastolic stress echocardiography: the time has come for its integration into clinical practice. J Am Soc Echocardiogr 2014; 27:1060–1063.
30. Paulus WJ, van Ballegoij JJM. Treatment of heart failure with normal ejection fraction: an inconvenient truth! J Am Coll Cardiol 2010; 55:526–537.
31. Wellens HJJ, Schwartz PJ, Lindemans FW, et al. Risk stratification for sudden cardiac death: current status and challenges for the future. Eur Heart J 2014; 35: 1642–1651.

32. Yusuf S, Pfeffer M, Swedberg et al. Effects of candesartan in patients with chronic heart failure and preserved left ventricular ejection fraction: the CHARM-PRESERVED trial. Lancet 2003; 362:777–81.

33. Flather M, Shibata M, Coats A, et al. Randomized trial to determine the effects of nebivolol on mortality and cardiovascular hospital admission in elderly patients with heart failure (SENIORS). Eur Heart J 2005; 26:215–225.
34. Ahmed A, Rich M, Fleg J, et al. Effects of digoxin on morbidity and mortality in diastolic heart failure: the ancillary digitalis investigation group trial. Circulation 2006; 114:397–403.
35. Cleland J, Tendera M, Adamus J, et al. The perindopril in elderly people with chronic heart failure (PEP-CHF) study. Eur Heart J 2006; 27:2338–2345.
36. Massie B, Carson P, McMurray J, et al. Irbesartan in patients with heart failure and preserved ejection fraction. New Engl J Med 2008; 359:2456–2467.
37. Solomon S, Zile M, Pieske B, et al. The angiotensin receptor neprilysin inhibitor LCZ696 in heart failure with preserved ejection fraction: a phase 2 double-blind randomised controlled trial. Lancet 2012; 380:1387–1395.
38. Edelman F, Wachter R, Schmidt A, et al. Effect of spironolactone on diastolic function and exercise capacity in patients with heart failure with preserved ejection fraction: the aldo-DHF randomized controlled trial. JAMA 2013; 309:781–791.
39. Redfield M, Chen H, Borlaug B, et al. Effect of phosphodiesterase-5 inhibition on exercise capacity and clinical status in heart failure with preserved ejection fraction: a randomized clinical trial. JAMA 2013; 309:1268–1277.
40. Pitt B, Pfeffer M, Assmann S, et al, Spironolactone for heart failure with preserved ejection fraction. New Engl J Med 2014; 370:1383–1392.

Chapter 9

Targeting BMPR-II deficiency for the treatment of pulmonary arterial hypertension

Mark L Ormiston, Nicholas W Morrell

PULMONARY ARTERIAL HYPERTENSION

Pulmonary arterial hypertension (PAH) is a subclassification of pulmonary hypertensive syndromes that is defined by a resting mean pulmonary artery pressure (PAP) at or above 25 mmHg in the absence of hypoxic lung disease, left heart disease, chronic thromboembolic pulmonary hypertension or other disorders known to cause elevated PAP (**Table 9.1**) [1]. PAH can arise as a primary disease, either in an idiopathic (IPAH) or heritable (HPAH) form, or can exist as a condition associated with immune disorders such as HIV, connective tissues diseases or exposure to particular drugs or toxins (**Table 9.2**). These disparate forms of PAH share a common pulmonary vascular pathology, characterised by medial thickening and the formation of occlusive vascular lesions that obstruct the pulmonary circulation at the level of the precapillary arterioles. This loss of the pulmonary microcirculation, and the resultant increase in pulmonary vascular resistance (PVR), leads to an elevation of PAP, right ventricular hypertrophy and often results in death due to right heart failure.

PAH is a rare disease, with a prevalence of 15–26 patients per million individuals and an incidence rate of 2.4–7.6 cases per million annually [2,3]. In its idiopathic and heritable

Table 9.1 Classification of pulmonary hypertension
1. Pulmonary arterial hypertension
2. Pulmonary hypertension due to left heart disease
3. Pulmonary hypertension due to lung diseases and/or hypoxia
4. Chronic thromboembolic pulmonary hypertension
5. Pulmonary hypertension with unclear multifactorial mechanisms
Adapted from Simonneau et al. [1].

Mark L Ormiston PhD, Department of Medicine, University of Cambridge School of Clinical Medicine, Addenbrooke's Hospital, Cambridge, UK

Nicholas W Morrell MD FRCP FMedSci, Department of Medicine, University of Cambridge School of Clinical Medicine, Addenbrooke's Hospital, Cambridge, UK. Email: nwm23@cam.ac.uk (for correspondence)

Class	Description
Table 9.2 Classification of pulmonary arterial hypertension [1]	
1.1	Idiopathic PAH
1.2	Heritable PAH:
1.2.1	*BMPR2*
1.2.2	*ALK-1, ENG, SMAD9, CAV1, KCNK3*
1.2.3	Unknown
1.3	Drug and toxin induced
1.4	Associated PAH with:
1.4.1	Connective tissue disease
1.4.2	HIV infection
1.3.3	Portal hypertension
1.4.4	Congenital heart diseases
1.4.5	Schistosomiasis
1'	Pulmonary veno-occlusive disease and/or pulmonary capillary haemangiomatosis
1"	Persistent pulmonary hypertension of the newborn

PAH, Pulmonary arterial hypertension.
From the 5th World Symposium on Pulmonary Hypertension (Nice, France, 2013).

forms, PAH presents in a relatively young patient population, aged 30–50 years, and preferentially in women at a rate of roughly 2:1. In addition to its relative infrequency, the diagnosis of PAH is complicated by the absence of symptoms in the early stages of disease. As a result, patients, typically, do not present in clinic until the disease has progressed to a more advanced state. From the French national PAH registry, the average mean PAP of patients at the time of diagnosis is 55 mmHg, with a mean PVR of >20 Woods units (equivalent to 160 MPa s/m^3) and a cardiac output of 2.5 L/min [2].

DISEASE PATHOLOGY

The classic vascular pathology observed in the lungs of patients with PAH is characterised by medial thickening, adventitial remodelling and the formation of intimal lesions that can be either laminar or nonlaminar in structure. These simple lesions, which are made of hyperproliferative myofibroblasts, smooth muscle cells (SMCs) and connective tissue matrix [4], are believed to account for a large component of elevated PVR in disease. Established PAH is also characterised by the formation of more complex, plexiform lesions. In plexiform lesions, a focal proliferation of clonal, apoptosis-resistant endothelial cells completely obliterates the lumen and can extend outside the vascular wall. The vessel is replaced by a series of narrow, endothelial-lined channels that are surrounded by myofibroblasts, SMCs and extracellular matrix components.

Although established PAH is associated with the rise of hyperproliferative endothelial cells and SMCs, the balance between endothelial cell proliferation and death remains a point of discussion in PAH. Work in both humans and animal models of disease has suggested that the initiation of PAH is associated with increased endothelial cell apoptosis.

Endothelial cells isolated from patients with PAH exhibit both increased proliferation and an enhanced susceptibility to apoptosis in response to various stimuli [5,6]. Furthermore, some of the most commonly used animal models of PAH, including the monocrotaline and Sugen-hypoxia rat models of disease, rely on pulmonary endothelial cell apoptosis as a critical step in their initiation [7,8].

In addition to vascular cell dysfunction, the pathogenesis of PAH is also associated with significant adventitial remodelling and perivascular inflammation. The adventitial enlargement observed in the lungs of patients with PAH is associated with extensive collagen deposition and the perivascular accumulation of T cells, B cells, mast cells, macrophages and dendritic cells, both infiltrating the vascular wall and within lesions [4]. In addition to these histopathological changes, previous studies have also identified an elevation of inflammatory cytokines, including TNF-α, interleukin (IL)-1β and IL-6 in the serum of IPAH and HPAH patients [9].

CURRENT TREATMENTS OF PAH

If left untreated, PAH will cause death by right-sided heart failure within 3–5 years of diagnosis. Fortunately, the last two decades have seen the approval of several new treatments of PAH that aim to reduce PVR through the stimulation of pulmonary vasodilation [10]. The regulation of vascular tone by endothelial cells and vascular SMCs is mediated by a balance of vasodilators, such as prostacyclin and nitric oxide (NO) and vasoconstrictive agents, including endothelin-1. Established PAH is associated with a shift in this balance towards excessive pulmonary vasoconstriction. Recognition of this imbalance was a driving force behind the approval of synthetic prostacyclin, or epoprostenol, for clinical use in 1996, and has since then resulted in a range of vasodilatory therapies that can be divided into three classes: (1) prostanoids, including epoprostenol and more stable prostacyclin analogues such as iloprost, beraprost and treprostinil; (2) endothelin receptor antagonists, including bosentan, ambrisentan and macitentan; and (3) phosphodiesterase-5 (PDE-5) inhibitors, such as sildenafil and tadalafil, which enhance vasodilation by prolonging the NO-mediated increase in cyclic guanosine monophosphate (**Figure 9.1**).

Despite the fact that these treatments have been shown to significantly extend patient survival from the time of diagnosis, improve their haemodynamic parameters and enhance their functional status, survival remains poor, with a 3-year survival rate of only 62% [11]. These treatments, which were originally intended as a bridge to lung transplantation, are also extremely expensive and, more importantly, do not capitalise on recent advances in our understanding of the molecular pathways that drive pathological vascular remodelling.

THE GENETIC BASIS OF PAH

Over the last 15 years, understanding of the pathobiology of PAH has been greatly enhanced by the identification of mutations in specific genes that are responsible for the heritable form of the disease. HPAH is an autosomal dominant disease, marked by a low penetrance (average 27%) of at-risk individuals [12]. While the existence of this familial form of PAH has been recognised since the first description of the disease, it was not until the year 2000 that two independent teams identified mutations in *BMPR2*, the gene encoding the bone morphogenetic protein (BMP) type II receptor (BMPR-II), as the cause

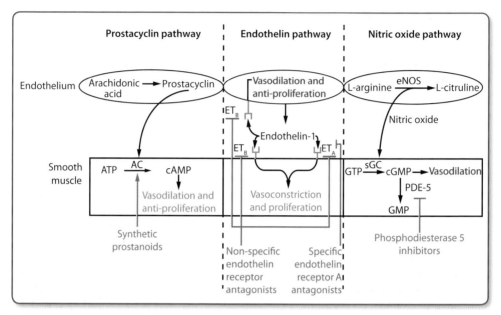

Figure 9.1 Current treatments of pulmonary arterial hypertension (PAH). Treatments of PAH target the prostacyclin, endothelin or nitric oxide pathways to enhance pulmonary vasodilation and block contraction and smooth muscle cell proliferation. AC, Adenylate cyclase; ATP, Adenosine triphosphate; cAMP, Cyclic adenosine monophosphate; cGMP: Cyclic guanosine monophosphate; ETA, Endothelin receptor A, ETB, Endothelin receptor B, eNOS, Endothelial nitric oxide synthase; GMP, Guanosine monophosphate; GTP, Guanosine triphosphate; PDE-5, Phosphodiesterase-5; sGC, Soluble guanylate cyclase.

of approximately 75% of HPAH cases [13,14]. Subsequent investigations have shown that *BMPR2* mutations also account for 15–26% of seemingly idiopathic cases of PAH, including both cases of de novo mutations and parental transmission with no record of a previous family history of disease. Considering the fact that IPAH is over 10 times more frequent than familial cases of disease, this means that the majority of PAH cases associated with *BMPR2* mutation occur in patients with no previous family history. In order to reflect this reality, the definition of HPAH was recently updated to include not only patients in a family with two or more documented cases of PAH, but also any patient with PAH possessing a mutation in *BMPR2*.

Since this initial discovery, over 400 different PAH-associated *BMPR2* mutations have been identified in all segments of the BMPR-II protein [12]. These include missense mutations within the extracellular domain, transmembrane region and intracellular kinase region, as well as nonsense mutations that encode premature termination codons (PTCs). Mutations in other genes associated with canonical BMPR-II-mediated signalling have also been shown to account for a small percentage of HPAH cases. These genes include *SMAD9*, which encodes the downstream transcription factor Smad8, as well as the BMP co-receptor endoglin (*ENG*) and the type I BMP receptor activin like receptor kinase-1 (Alk1, gene symbol *ACVRL1*). Both *ENG* and *ACVRL1* mutations are primarily associated with hereditary haemorrhagic telangectasia (HHT), a disease that causes vascular abnormalities, including telangetectasias in the skin and mucosal regions, and arteriovenous malformations in the lung, liver and brain. Importantly, while *ACVRL1* and

ENG-related cases of HHT are occasionally associated with PAH, these mutations have not been shown to cause PAH in the absence of HHT.

More recently, the application of advanced genomic screening technologies has allowed for the identification of rare mutations in other genes that are responsible for a small fraction of HPAH and IPAH cases. These include mutations in the gene *KCNK3*, which encodes the acid-sensitive potassium channel TASK-1 [15], and *CAV1*, which encodes the protein caveolin-1, a main component of the caveolae lipid rafts in cell membranes [16]. A genome-wide association study has also identified common variants of *CBLN2*, the gene for cerebellin-2, that are associated with a predisposition towards the development of PAH. Despite the fact that mutations in these genes account for only a small fraction of the PAH patient population, the identification of each new gene brings with it an enhanced understanding of the cell signalling pathways that are critically altered during the development of PAH.

In contrast, *BMPR2* mutations account for roughly 25% of all IPAH and HPAH cases. Patients bearing *BMPR2* mutations develop PAH earlier; have more severe disease; and die sooner than those without mutations [17]. Interestingly, patients with PAH with *BMPR2* mutations exhibit reductions in BMPR-II protein levels of >75% when compared to control subjects, suggesting that the development of PAH can suppress receptor levels to a degree that is greater than what can be accounted for by haploinsufficiency alone [17]. Reduced BMPR-II protein levels and impaired downstream signalling have also been identified in patients with IPAH lacking mutations in *BMPR2*, as well as in common, nongenetic rodent models of disease [18], further supporting a central role for reduced BMPR-II signalling in most forms of the disease, independent of aetiology. When taken together, these factors make the BMPR-II signalling pathway an extremely attractive target for next-generation therapeutic intervention. Some of the most promising strategies currently being investigated for enhancing BMPR-II signalling in PAH (**Figure 9.2**) are described below.

ADMINISTRATION OF BMPR-II AGONISTS

Exogenous BMP ligands

The most direct strategy for targeting BMPR-II deficiency in PAH involves the delivery of exogenous BMP ligand to enhance signalling via the remaining functional receptor. Proof-of-concept studies using patient-derived pulmonary artery SMCs (PASMCs) have shown that the addition of increasing concentrations of BMP ligand can overcome the functional defects associated with *BMPR2* mutation in vitro [19]. However, the translation of this strategy into in vivo preclinical studies has been limited by uncertainty regarding which cell type or types are critical to the initiation and progression of pathological vascular remodelling.

Following the initial identification of *BMPR2* mutation in PAH, much of the work investigating the role this receptor in disease pathogenesis focussed on the impact of these mutations on PASMC proliferation and migration. PASMCs from BMPR-II mutation carriers have been shown to exhibit a more proliferative phenotype and insensitivity to the antiproliferative effects of specific BMPs and transforming growth factor-β (TGF-β) [19]. However, later studies also examined a role for impaired endothelial BMP signalling in the pathogenesis of PAH. In addition to increased endothelial cell proliferation and enhanced susceptibility to apoptosis [5,6], loss of BMPR-II has also been shown to influence endothelial cell barrier integrity and pulmonary vascular leak [20]. It has also

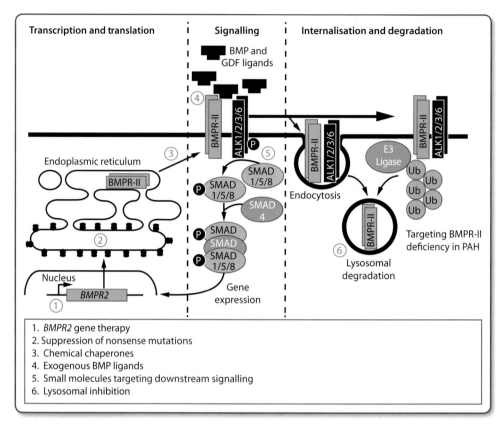

Figure 9.2 Strategies for targeting bone morphogenetic protein type II receptor deficiency in the treatment of pulmonary arterial hypertension. BMP, Bone morphogenetic protein; BMPR-II, Bone morphogenetic protein type II receptor; GDF, growth differentiation factor.

been suggested that *BMPR2* mutations can impact on other cell types that may contribute to disease pathology, including effects on cardiomyocyte hypertrophy in response to increased right ventricular load [21], as well as a potential role for *BMPR2* mutation in immune cell dysfunction [9].

Identifying the appropriate BMP ligand to selectively target cell types of interest also presents a significant challenge. BMPs are members of the TGF-β superfamily, a highly complex family of proteins including over 30 ligands that signal through heteromeric complexes of type I and type II receptors. As a type II receptor of this superfamily, BMPR-II can form complexes with several type I receptors, including Alk1, Alk2, Alk3 or Alk6, with each receptor complex recognising a specific subset of BMP ligands [22]. Although the downstream effects of signalling via BMPR-II are greatly influenced by the components making up this ligand–receptor complex, canonical signalling generally involves phosphorylation of the Smad-1, 5 or -8 transcription factors, which complex with the co-smad, Smad-4, and translocate to the nucleus to induce gene expression (**Figure 9.2**). BMP signalling is also regulated by a number of accessory receptors, including endoglin, which further enhance the ligand- and tissue-specific nature of BMP responses.

Fortunately, when considering the therapeutic delivery of exogenous BMPs, recent studies describing disease phenotypes associated with mutations in type I receptors, and knowledge of the tissue-specific distribution of these proteins, can be used to inform decisions. In smooth muscle, BMP ligands, including BMP2 and BMP4, block serum-induced proliferation via complexes of BMPR-II with Alk3 or Alk6 [19]. However, mutations in *ALK3* and *ALK6* do not cause pulmonary vascular disease, but are, instead, associated with juvenile gastrointestinal polyposis [23] and hereditary brachydactyly [24], respectively. This fact calls into question the importance of these receptors, and the signalling complexes that they form, in the pathogenesis of PAH. In contrast, the reported development of PAH in HHT patients bearing mutations in the genes encoding Alk1 or endoglin indicates that the receptor complexes formed by these molecules are somehow involved in the maintenance of pulmonary vascular homeostasis. Interestingly, both Alk1 and endoglin are found almost exclusively on the endothelium, suggesting that any therapeutic ligand should target pulmonary endothelial cells.

Although Alk1 was originally thought to be an orphan receptor, a 2007 study identified BMP9 and BMP10 as ligands that signal via complexes of Alk1 with either BMPR-II or ActRII [25]. Endoglin has also been shown to interact with Alk1/BMPR-II complexes, as well as an alternative TGF-β receptor complex containing Alk1, Alk5 and TGF-bR-II [22]. Based on this information, we have recently examined the therapeutic delivery of BMP9 to target endothelial dysfunction in PAH. In vitro, BMP9 prevents the enhanced apoptosis observed in *BMPR2* mutation-bearing endothelial cells and promotes monolayer integrity through the formation of tight junctions. In vivo, BMP prevents and reverses established disease in a range of rodent models, including spontaneous disease in a mouse model bearing a knock-in of the PAH-associated *R899X–BMPR2* mutation (unpublished results).

One concern associated with the delivery of exogenous BMP ligands is off target effects, such as the undesirable calcification of soft tissues that has been reported in response to exogenous BMP9 overexpression [26]. While no such calcification was observed in the work detailed above, future studies may examine the use of genetically modified BMP ligands that maximise the beneficial effects on endothelial survival and vascular integrity, while minimising the capacity of these ligands to stimulate bone formation.

Small-molecule BMPR-II agonists

One alternative to the direct administration of BMP ligand involves the use of small molecules that either agonise BMPR-II or enhance downstream BMP signalling. We have previously shown that prostanoids and sildenafil, both currently licensed for the treatment of PAH, exert beneficial effects on BMP/Smad signalling, as well as downstream Inhibitor of DNA-binding protein 1 (*ID1*) gene expression, and can partly restore signalling in PASMCs bearing *BMPR2* mutations (**Figure 9.3**) [27,28]. In animal models of PAH associated with reduced expression of BMPR-II, iloprost or sildenafil increases Smad/*ID1* signalling in pulmonary arteries and prevents the development of PAH.

Another recent study exploring this treatment strategy used high throughput screening of 3756 US Food and Drug Administration approved compounds to identify molecules that enhanced the activity of BMP-responsive elements of the promoter for *ID1* [29]. Among the top drug candidates emerging from this screen was Tacrolimus (FK506). FK506 is an immunosuppressive drug that acts in T cells by binding the FK-binding protein-12 (FKBP12). This complex inhibits calcineurin, thereby blocking the dephosphorylation of the nuclear factor of activated T cells and preventing the transcription of IL-2. FKBP12

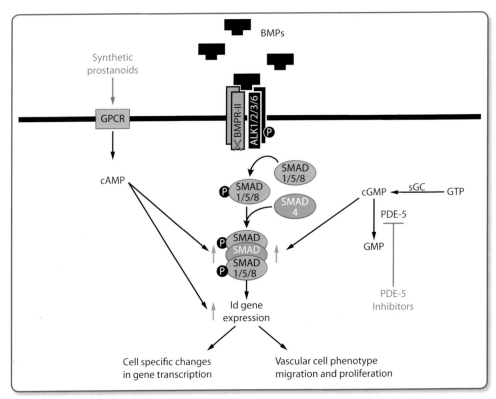

Figure 9.3 Influence of existing pulmonary arterial hypertension (PAH) therapies on bone morphogenetic protein type II receptor (BMPR-II) signalling and cell phenotype. Existing treatments of PAH, including synthetic prostanoids and phosphodiesterase-5 (PDE-5) inhibitors interact with and enhance canonical BMPR-II signalling and downstream Id gene expression. BMP, Bone morphogenetic protein; cAMP, Cyclic adenosine monophosphate; cGMP: Cyclic guanosine monophosphate; GMP, guanosine monophosphate; GPCR; GTP, Guanosine triphosphate; sGC, Soluble guanylate cyclase.

has also been shown to bind to type I receptors and inhibit BMP signalling by serving as a docking protein for calcineurin. It has been proposed that FK506 potentiates BMPR-II-mediated signalling in endothelial cells by the dual actions of releasing FKBP12 from type I receptors and inhibiting calcineurin. FK506 was found to rescue dysfunctional BMP signalling in endothelial cells from patients with PAH with *BMPR2* mutations and reversed established disease in multiple rodent models of PAH. Early clinical trials are currently underway to establish the viability of this strategy as a treatment of PAH.

RESCUING MUTANT BMPR-II RECEPTOR FUNCTION

Therapeutic strategies for enhancing BMPR-II-mediated signalling can be achieved through multiple approaches. In addition to targeting residual cell surface BMPR-II with ligands or small molecules, alternative approaches have included strategies designed to enhance BMP signalling by rescuing the mutated copy of the *BMPR2* gene. These strategies vary depending on the type of mutation present. Missense mutations encoding misfolded but functionally active BMPR-II can be targeted with chemical chaperones that enhance the transport of the mutant protein to the cell surface. Alternatively, alleles bearing nonsense mutations can be targeted with compounds that promote the translational read-through of PTCs. Both approaches have greatly benefited from extensive preclinical and clinical research in cystic fibrosis, where both missense and nonsense mutations in the cystic fibrosis transmembrane conductance regulator (CFTR) have been targeted for rescue.

Chemical chaperones

Of the known PAH-associated mutations in *BMPR2*, roughly 30% consist of missense mutations in functionally important domains of the receptor. These mutations do not only impact on receptor activation but have also been shown to influence protein processing and trafficking to the cell surface. In particular, mutations involving the substitution of cysteine residues within both the extracellular and kinase domains of BMPR-II have been shown to cause improper folding of the protein, retention in the endoplasmic reticulum (ER) and reduced trafficking to the cell surface [30]. Not only does this retention reduce the amount of cell surface BMPR-II that is available for ligand binding, but certain missense mutations, particularly the *C118W* cysteine substitution in the extracellular domain, have also been shown to exert a dominant negative effect by causing co-retention of type I receptors within the ER.

Strategies for enhancing the processing and cell-surface trafficking of mutant proteins have focussed on the use of compounds known as 'chemical chaperones', which aim to either promote proper protein folding or facilitate the release of misfolded, but functionally active protein from the ER. Under normal physiological conditions, chaperone proteins within the ER stabilise newly synthesised proteins, prevent their aggregation and promote folding. When a mutation is present that prevents correct protein folding or recognition, these chaperones also make up a quality control mechanism that retains misfolded proteins within the ER and targets them for degradation via the proteasome.

Some chemical chaperones, such as glycerol, nonselectively stabilise the tertiary structure of the mutant proteins and facilitate folding. Other compounds, including thapsigargin and sodium 4-phenylbutyrate (4-PBA), inhibit the interactions of the mutant protein with the chaperone proteins responsible for their recognition, retention and degradation. Thapsigargin is a sarcoplasmic or endoplasmic reticulum calcium ATPase (SERCA) calcium pump inhibitor that depletes calcium stores within the ER, facilitating the release of retained proteins from chaperone proteins that rely on the elevated concentration of calcium ions within the ER for their activity. In contrast, 4-PBA enhances misfolded protein release by reducing the expression of the chaperone hsc70 [31]. In cystic fibrosis, 4-PBA has been shown to rescue chloride channel function by facilitating the trafficking of the misfolded *F508del* CFTR mutant protein to the cell surface. Randomised control trials exploring the use of 4-PBA in cystic fibrosis have also produced promising results [32].

Chemical chaperones have also been investigated for PAH, where a panel of compounds, including 4-PBA, glycerol and thapsigargin, were shown to promote trafficking of *C118W* BMPR-II protein to the cell surface and restore downstream Smad signalling [33]. While these results are promising, there are several factors limiting the clinical application of these compounds for PAH. Unlike in cystic fibrosis, where *F508del* is the most common disease causing mutation, the PAH patient population contains a large variety of missense mutations, only a subset of which encode functionally active receptors. As a result, translation of this treatment strategy into the clinic is likely to be complicated by fact that these various mutations are not only rare, but are also likely to exhibit differential responsiveness to chemical chaperone treatment.

Suppression of nonsense mutations

In addition to missense mutations, nonsense mutations encoding PTCs also make up roughly 30% of the known PAH-associated mutations in *BMPR2*. The mRNA transcripts produced by these alleles are typically subject to nonsense-mediated decay, resulting in reduced *BMPR2* mRNA and decreased protein levels. Unlike missense mutations, where the mutant protein is targeted for rescue, the treatment of nonsense mutations requires the use of compounds that suppress or silence PTCs, allowing for the translation of mutant mRNA into full-length, functional protein [34].

Of the various compounds that have been shown to induce PTC read-through, the best characterised belong to the aminoglycoside family of antibiotics. Aminoglycosides bind to the decoding centre of prokaryotic ribosomal RNA, which monitors base pairing between codons and anticodons and is thus responsible for the maintenance of translational fidelity. In bacteria, aminoglycosides cause a reduction in this translational proofreading at low doses and completely block translational initiation at higher doses.

A diminished binding affinity of aminoglycosides for the mammalian decoding centre has allowed for dosing ranges that enable antimicrobial function in humans without impacting on protein synthesis. However, a number of aminoglycosides, including gentamicin, G418 and streptomycin, have been shown to weakly bind the eukaryotic decoding centre. At high doses, these compounds induce read-through of PTCs in mammalian cells without causing the misreading of sense codons. A wide range of aminoglycosides has been shown to suppress disease-causing PTCs and partially restore protein function in nonsense mutation-bearing cell culture models of multiple diseases, including cystic fibrosis, Duchenne muscular dystrophy and PAH [35]. Clinical trials exploring the administration of gentamicin to patients carrying nonsense mutations with cystic fibrosis and other diseases have also demonstrated the ability of these compounds to induce the partial restoration of full-length, functional protein. However, the high doses required to achieve these beneficial effects are also associated with renal toxicity and hearing loss, thus preventing the widespread use of aminoglycosides in clinical applications.

Ongoing work is aiming to minimise the off-target effects of aminoglycosides through the selective production of specific gentamicin isomers or the generation of aminoglycoside derivatives that improve PTC suppression while minimising off-target effects. More recently, high-throughput screens have identified other compounds distinct from aminoglycosides that possess the ability to effectively suppress PTCs without affecting the recognition of normal stop signals. One such compound, the small molecule ataluren (PTC124), is currently in phase III clinical trials for cystic fibrosis. In PAH, ataluren was shown to increase BMPR-II protein levels and downstream signalling in primary cells from patients with nonsense mutations in *BMPR2* and *SMAD9* [36]. These effects were accompanied by a restoration of normal proliferation rates in hyperproliferative, patient-derived pulmonary arterial endothelial cells and PASMCs.

ENHANCING BMPR-II EXPRESSION

Inhibition of lysosomal degradation

A third approach that has been explored for enhancing BMP signalling involves extending the longevity of BMPR-II at the cell surface. This approach requires an understanding of the kinetics of BMPR-II turnover in vascular cells and the methods by which the receptor is internalised and degraded. Previous work by our group has shown that BMPR-II is rapidly turned over in endothelial cells, with notable protein loss reported as early as 1 hour following the blockade of new protein synthesis [37]. This finding is consistent with the report that BMPR-II is subjected to constitutive endocytosis by both clathirin and caveolae-mediated pathways [38]. Additional work has shown that BMPR-II can also be targeted for ubiquitination by Kaposi's sarcoma herpes virus K5 E3 ligase, and directed for lysosomal degradation [39]. Each of these findings highlights the lysosome as the primary route for BMPR-II turnover and points to lysosomal inhibition as a promising target for preserving BMPR-II longevity and enhancing receptor-mediated signalling.

Several compounds can achieve lysosomal inhibition, largely through the prevention of vesicular acidification. Concanamycin A (Con-A), which blocks acidification through the inhibition of vacuolar ATPases, has been shown to increase endogenous BMPR-II protein levels in endothelial cells [37]. However, Con-A has no effect on receptor internalisation, resulting in the accumulation of BMPR-II protein in inactive lysosomes, not at the cell surface where it can enhance signalling. Furthermore, Con-A is highly toxic, making it unsuitable for clinical use.

An alternative approach for lysosomal inhibition is the 4-aminoquinolone, chloroquine. Used for decades as a prophylactic antimalarial drug, chloroquine and its less toxic derivative hydroxychloroquine have recently been repurposed for use in the treatment of rheumatoid arthritis and cancer. Chloroquine is a weak, lipophilic base, which passes freely through cell membranes. Upon entry into the acidic lysosome ($pH \sim 4.6$) chloroquine is protonated, preventing diffusion out and resulting in lysosomal accumulation, elevated pH and lysosomal inactivation. Importantly, chloroquine also has well-documented effects on molecules involved in endocytic degradation. Accumulation of chloroquine in the lysosome inhibits phospholipase A2, which is critical to multiple endocytic pathways, providing a mechanism other than lysosomal inhibition by which it can preserve BMPR-II at the cell surface [40].

As with Con-A, chloroquine can enhance BMPR-II protein levels in endothelial cells. However, unlike Con-A, which only blocked lysosomal degradation, pharmacologically relevant concentrations of chloroquine also increased cell surface BMPR-II and rescued the expression of downstream signalling targets such as *ID1* in *BMPR2* mutation-bearing endothelial cells [37]. The ability of chloroquine to promote BMPR-II at the cell surface in addition to accumulation in the lysosomes highlights the broad-acting nature of this compound. Beyond its direct effect on BMPR-II, other studies have attributed the therapeutic benefit of chloroquine in PAH to an inhibition of autophagy. Autophagy is the process of 'self-eating', whereby defective or surplus cellular components are enclosed in an intracellular vesicle known as an autophagosome, which fuses with a lysosome to enact degradation and recycling. By inhibiting lysosomal acidification, chloroquine targets the final stage of the autophagy pathway. While autophagy is a normal process in healthy cells, rapidly proliferating cells, such as tumour cells or the aberrantly proliferative vacular cells in the lesions of patients with PAH, can become reliant on autophagy for survival. By blocking autophagy, chloroquine can cause these cells to undergo apoptosis, providing yet another pathway by which this compound can provide therapeutic benefit.

In vivo, both chloroquine and hydroxychloroquine inhibited the development of pulmonary hypertension and blocked the progression of established disease in the monocrotaline rat model [41]. This action was associated with the inhibition of several components of the autophagy pathway, as well as the preservation of BMPR-II protein levels, which are decreased in monocrotaline-treated rats. Importantly, this effect was achieved with minimal effect on *BMPR2* mRNA expression, highlighting the ability of chloroquine to enhance BMPR-II mediated signalling by preserving receptor longevity.

Translation of hydroxychloroquine into a clinical therapy is facilitated by the fact that the compound is inexpensive and presents minimal toxicity or side effects at therapeutically effective doses. Long-term treatment with hydroxychloroquine has been associated with retinopathy in 0.5–1% of patients. However, this result can be avoided with proper monitoring of patients undergoing treatment.

BMPR2 gene therapy

Gene therapy techniques have also been explored in animal models of PAH as a means to restore BMPR-II receptor levels. The targeted delivery of an adenoviral vector containing the *BMPR2* gene to the pulmonary vascular endothelium of rats substantially reduced the severity of pulmonary hypertension in the chronic hypoxia and monocrotaline models of PAH [42,43]. For these studies, targeting of the adenoviral vectors to the pulmonary endothelium appeared to be a key feature of therapeutic efficacy, as similar studies targeting the pulmonary vascular smooth muscle using aerosol vector delivery failed to demonstrate any measurable benefit in the monocrotaline rat model.

CONCLUSION

Identification of the link between PAH and BMPR-II haploinsufficiency has provided considerable insight into the pathogenesis of disease, as well as the molecular mechanisms governing pulmonary vascular homeostasis. This discovery also provides an ideal candidate pathway for proof-of-concept studies involving targeted pharmacological therapies that aim to treat disease through enhancing BMPR-II-mediated signalling. In the 15 years since the identification of *BMPR2* mutations in patients with PAH, considerable work has gone into clarifying the relevant cell types and signalling pathways that connect *BMPR2* mutation to disease pathogenesis and have identified the pulmonary endothelium as a key factor in these processes. Ongoing studies will aim to capitalise on this work to translate proof-of-concept studies in preclinical animal models to viable treatments in patients.

Key points for clinical practice

- PAH is a disease of occlusive vascular remodelling.
- Existing vasodilatory therapies do not address the underlying factors driving disease pathology.
- Mutations in BMPR2, the gene encoding the BMPR-II, are responsible for approximately 25% of PAH cases.
- Reduced BMPR-II is also observed in patients with PAH lacking mutations.
- Therapeutic strategies targeting BMPR-II deficiency can involve (1) the stimulation of canonical receptor signalling, (2) rescue of mutant receptor transcription and translation or (3) enhancement of receptor expression and longevity.

REFERENCES

1. Simonneau G, Gatzoulis MA, Adatia I, et al. Updated clinical classification of pulmonary hypertension. J Am Coll Cardiol 2013; 62:D34–D41. PubMed PMID: 24355639.
2. Humbert M, Sitbon O, Chaouat A, et al. Pulmonary arterial hypertension in France: results from a national registry. Am J Respir Crit Care Med 2006; 173:1023–1030. PubMed PMID: 16456139.
3. Peacock AJ, Murphy NF, McMurray JJ, Caballero L, Stewart S. An epidemiological study of pulmonary arterial hypertension. Eur Respir J 2007; 30:104–109. PubMed PMID: 17360728.
4. Tuder RM, Marecki JC, Richter A, Fijalkowska I, Flores S. Pathology of pulmonary hypertension. Clin Chest Med 2007; 28:23–42, vii. PubMed PMID: 17338926.
5. Toshner M, Voswinckel R, Southwood M, et al. Evidence of dysfunction of endothelial progenitors in pulmonary arterial hypertension. Am J Respir Crit Care Med 2009; 180:780–787. PubMed PMID: 19628780. Epub 2009/07/25. eng.
6. Lavoie JR, Ormiston ML, Perez-Iratxeta C, et al. Proteomic analysis implicates translationally controlled tumor protein as a novel mediator of occlusive vascular remodeling in pulmonary arterial hypertension. Circulation 2014; 129:2125–2135. PubMed PMID: 24657995.
7. Wilson DW, Segall HJ, Pan LC, et al. Mechanisms and pathology of monocrotaline pulmonary toxicity. Crit Rev Toxicol 1992; 22:307–325. PubMed PMID: 1489509.
8. Taraseviciene-Stewart L, Kasahara Y, Alger L, et al. Inhibition of the VEGF receptor 2 combined with chronic hypoxia causes cell death-dependent pulmonary endothelial cell proliferation and severe pulmonary hypertension. Faseb J 2001; 15:427–438. PubMed PMID: 11156958.
9. Rabinovitch M, Guignabert C, Humbert M, Nicolls MR. Inflammation and immunity in the pathogenesis of pulmonary arterial hypertension. Circ Res 2014; 115:165–175. PubMed PMID: 24951765. Pubmed Central PMCID: 4097142.
10. Seferian A, Simonneau G. Therapies for pulmonary arterial hypertension: where are we today, where do we go tomorrow? Eur Respir Rev 2013; 22:217–226. PubMed PMID: 23997048.
11. National Audit of Pulmonary Hypertension. Leeds, UK: Health and Social Care Information Centre, 2013.
12. Austin ED, Loyd JE. The genetics of pulmonary arterial hypertension. Circ Res 2014; 115:189–202. PubMed PMID: 24951767. Pubmed Central PMCID: 4137413.
13. Lane KB, Machado RD, Pauciulo MW, et al. Heterozygous germline mutations in BMPR2, encoding a TGF-beta receptor, cause familial primary pulmonary hypertension. The International PPH Consortium. Nat Genet 2000; 26:81–84. PubMed PMID: 10973254.
14. Deng Z, Morse JH, Slager SL, et al. Familial primary pulmonary hypertension (gene PPH1) is caused by mutations in the bone morphogenetic protein receptor-II gene. Am J Hum Genet 2000; 67:737–744. PubMed PMID: 10903931.
15. Ma L, Roman-Campos D, Austin ED, et al. A novel channelopathy in pulmonary arterial hypertension. N Engl J Med 2013; 369:351–361. PubMed PMID: 23883380. Pubmed Central PMCID: 3792227.
16. Austin ED, Ma L, LeDuc C, et al. Whole exome sequencing to identify a novel gene (caveolin-1) associated with human pulmonary arterial hypertension. Circ Cardiovasc Genet 2012; 5:336–343. PubMed PMID: 22474227. Pubmed Central PMCID: 3380156.
17. Atkinson C, Stewart S, Upton PD, et al. Primary pulmonary hypertension is associated with reduced pulmonary vascular expression of type II bone morphogenetic protein receptor. Circulation 2002; 105:1672–1728. PubMed PMID: 11940546.
18. Long L, Crosby A, Yang X, et al. Altered bone morphogenetic protein and transforming growth factor-beta signaling in rat models of pulmonary hypertension: potential for activin receptor-like kinase-5 inhibition in prevention and progression of disease. Circulation 2009; 119:566–576. PubMed PMID: 19153267. Epub 2009/01/21. eng.
19. Yang J, Davies RJ, Southwood M, et al. Mutations in bone morphogenetic protein type II receptor cause dysregulation of Id gene expression in pulmonary artery smooth muscle cells: implications for familial pulmonary arterial hypertension. Circ Res 2008; 102:1212–1221. PubMed PMID: 18436795. Epub 2008/04/26. eng.
20. Burton VJ, Ciuclan LI, Holmes AM, et al. Bone morphogenetic protein receptor II regulates pulmonary artery endothelial cell barrier function. Blood 2011; 117:333–341. PubMed PMID: 20724539.
21. Hemnes AR, Brittain EL, Trammell AW, et al. Evidence for right ventricular lipotoxicity in heritable pulmonary arterial hypertension. Am J Respir Crit Care Med 201 2014; 189:325–334.

22. Upton PD, Morrell NW. TGF-beta and BMPR-II pharmacology – implications for pulmonary vascular diseases. Curr Opin Pharmacol 2009; 9:274–280. PubMed PMID: 19321386. Epub 2009/03/27. eng.

23. Howe JR, Bair JL, Sayed MG, et al. Germline mutations of the gene encoding bone morphogenetic protein receptor 1A in juvenile polyposis. Nat Genet 2001; 28:184–187. PubMed PMID: 11381269.

24. Lehmann K, Seemann P, Stricker S, et al. Mutations in bone morphogenetic protein receptor 1B cause brachydactyly type A2. Proc Natl Acad Sci USA 2003; 100:12277–12282. PubMed PMID: 14523231. Pubmed Central PMCID: 218749.

25. David L, Mallet C, Mazerbourg S, Feige JJ, Bailly S. Identification of BMP9 and BMP10 as functional activators of the orphan activin receptor-like kinase 1 (ALK1) in endothelial cells. Blood 2007; 109:1953–1961. PubMed PMID: 17068149.

26. Kang Q, Sun MH, Cheng H, et al. Characterization of the distinct orthotopic bone-forming activity of 14 BMPs using recombinant adenovirus-mediated gene delivery. Gene Ther 2004; 11:1312–1320. PubMed PMID: 15269709.

27. Yang J, Li X, Al-Lamki RS, et al. Smad-dependent and smad-independent induction of id1 by prostacyclin analogues inhibits proliferation of pulmonary artery smooth muscle cells in vitro and in vivo. Circ Res 2010; 107:252–262. PubMed PMID: 20522807.

28. Yang J, Li X, Al-Lamki RS, et al. Sildenafil potentiates bone morphogenetic protein signaling in pulmonary arterial smooth muscle cells and in experimental pulmonary hypertension. Arterioscler Thromb Vasc Biol 2013; 33:34–42. PubMed PMID: 23139294.

29. Spiekerkoetter E, Tian X, Cai J, et al. FK506 activates BMPR2, rescues endothelial dysfunction, and reverses pulmonary hypertension. J Clin Invest 2013; 123:3600–3613. PubMed PMID: 23867624. Pubmed Central PMCID: 3726153.

30. Rudarakanchana N, Flanagan JA, Chen H, et al. Functional analysis of bone morphogenetic protein type II receptor mutations underlying primary pulmonary hypertension. Hum Mol Genet 2002; 11:1517–1525. PubMed PMID: 12045205.

31. Rubenstein RC, Zeitlin PL. Sodium 4-phenylbutyrate downregulates Hsc70: implications for intracellular trafficking of DeltaF508-CFTR. Am J Physiol Cell Physiol 2000; 278:C259–C267. PubMed PMID: 10666020.

32. Rubenstein RC, Zeitlin PL. A pilot clinical trial of oral sodium 4-phenylbutyrate (Buphenyl) in deltaF508-homozygous cystic fibrosis patients: partial restoration of nasal epithelial CFTR function. Am J Respir Crit Care Med 1998; 157:484–490. PubMed PMID: 9476862.

33. Sobolewski A, Rudarakanchana N, Upton PD, et al. Failure of bone morphogenetic protein receptor trafficking in pulmonary arterial hypertension: potential for rescue. Hum Mol Genet 2008;17:3180–3190. PubMed PMID: 18647753.

34. Keeling KM, Bedwell DM. Suppression of nonsense mutations as a therapeutic approach to treat genetic diseases. Wiley Interdiscip Rev RNA 2011; 2:837–852. PubMed PMID: 21976286. Pubmed Central PMCID: 3188951.

35. Nasim MT, Ghouri A, Patel B, et al. Stoichiometric imbalance in the receptor complex contributes to dysfunctional BMPR-II mediated signalling in pulmonary arterial hypertension. Hum Mol Genet 2008; 17:1683–1694. PubMed PMID: 18321866.

36. Drake KM, Dunmore BJ, McNelly LN, Morrell NW, Aldred MA. Correction of nonsense BMPR2 and SMAD9 mutations by ataluren in pulmonary arterial hypertension. Am J Respir Cell Mol Biol 2013; 49:403–409. PubMed PMID: 23590310. Pubmed Central PMCID: 3824059.

37. Dunmore BJ, Drake KM, Upton PD, et al. The lysosomal inhibitor, chloroquine, increases cell surface BMPR-II levels and restores BMP9 signalling in endothelial cells harbouring BMPR-II mutations. Hum Mol Genet 2013; 22:3667–3679. PubMed PMID: 23669347. Pubmed Central PMCID: 3749859.

38. Hartung A, Bitton-Worms K, Rechtman MM, et al. Different routes of bone morphogenic protein (BMP) receptor endocytosis influence BMP signaling. Mol Cell Biol 2006; 26:7791–7805. PubMed PMID: 16923969. Pubmed Central PMCID: 1636853.

39. Durrington HJ, Upton PD, Hoer S, et al. Identification of a lysosomal pathway regulating degradation of the bone morphogenetic protein receptor type II. J Biol Chem 2010; 285:37641–37649. PubMed PMID: 20870717. Pubmed Central PMCID: 2988369.

40. Doody AM, Antosh AL, Brown WJ. Cytoplasmic phospholipase A2 antagonists inhibit multiple endocytic membrane trafficking pathways. Biochem Biophys Res Commun 2009; 388:695–699. PubMed PMID: 19695219. Pubmed Central PMCID: 2764267.

41. Long L, Yang X, Southwood M, et al. Chloroquine prevents progression of experimental pulmonary hypertension via inhibition of autophagy and lysosomal bone morphogenetic protein type II receptor degradation. Circ Res 2013;112:1159–1170. PubMed PMID: 23446737.

42. Reynolds AM, Xia W, Holmes MD, et al. Bone morphogenetic protein type 2 receptor gene therapy attenuates hypoxic pulmonary hypertension. Am J Physiol Lung Cell Mol Physiol 2007; 292:L1182–L1192. PubMed PMID: 17277049.

43. Reynolds AM, Holmes MD, Danilov SM, Reynolds PN. Targeted gene delivery of BMPR2 attenuates pulmonary hypertension. Eur Respir J 2012; 39:329–343. PubMed PMID: 21737550.

Chapter 10

Inappropriate sinus tachycardia

Brian Olshansky, Renee M Sullivan

INTRODUCTION

Sinus tachycardia is ubiquitous, expected and, in appropriate circumstances normal. In most instances, the cause can be explained by parasympathetic withdrawal and/or sympathetic activation due to physical activity, psychological stress, ingested substances or drugs and a multitude of medical conditions (**Table 10.1**). For some individuals, sinus tachycardia cannot be explained by physiological demands, and may happen at rest, with minimal exertion, or during recovery from exercise. Patients with this type of tachycardia are said to have inappropriate sinus tachycardia (IST), which is the focus of this chapter.

DEFINITION OF IST

While the definition remains in dispute and the condition is obscure, the IST syndrome is an otherwise unexplained sinus tachycardia, rate over 100 bpm consistently or intermittently at rest and/or a sinus rate that accelerates excessively with, or remains fast, even with minimal exercise. Some include in this definition an average heart rate over 24 hours exceeding 90 bpm. Critical to this definition is the presence of associated, sometimes debilitating, symptoms. The definition is overall complex; many individuals may be considered to have IST but if symptoms are not present or sinus tachycardia is only occasional, the diagnosis of this syndrome cannot be made.

Table 10.1 Causes of appropriate sinus tachycardia	
'Routine' causes	Exercise, anxiety, pain
Medical conditions	Anaemia, dehydration, pulmonary embolus, fever, pericarditis, aortic insufficiency, mitral insufficiency, myocardial infarction, pulmonary oedema, pneumothorax, hyperthyroidism, hypoglycaemia
Drugs and interventions	Anticholinergics, catecholamines, alcohol, caffeine, cocaine, tobacco, beta-blocker withdrawal, AV nodal slow pathway ablation (for AVNRT)
AV, atrioventricular; AVNRT, atrioventricular nodal re-entry tachycardia.	

Brian Olshansky MD, Covance, Princeton, NJ, USA. Email: brian-olshansky@uiowa.edu (for correspondence)

Renee M Sullivan MD, Covance, Princeton, NJ, USA.

CLINICAL PRESENTATION

Typically, the patient with IST is a young, otherwise healthy, woman bothered with palpitations and rapid heartbeat along with dizziness, fatigue, weakness and various nonspecific complaints. For some individuals, sinus tachycardia can itself be highly symptomatic or be associated with a constellation of symptoms that may, or may not, be related directly to the tachycardia itself, thus leading the individual to present himself or herself to a physician for further evaluation and potential treatments. While symptoms in IST may be severe, the prognosis is generally benign, perhaps, in part, due to the fluctuation of heart rate represented by a diurnal variation [1] in distinct contrast to the prognosis in tachycardia-mediated cardiomyopathy in which the heart rate is rarely controlled and may not decrease at night. 'Deconditioning' must be distinguished from IST. Non-IST arrhythmias can also coexist with IST [2].

Most patients with IST are otherwise healthy without comorbidities. In fact, almost any other comorbidity that is present must be suspected as the cause for the tachycardia. As IST appears to be common in healthcare providers, surreptitious use of stimulants and drugs, such as insulin, amphetamines, caffeine or other substances, must be considered.

A psychological disorder is often present in IST; its relationship to tachycardia is uncertain. One report indicates 100% of patients with IST had some form of psychiatric disorder (schizophrenia, depression, panic disorder or somatoform disorder [3]). Patients with IST tend to deny that psychiatric issues are present. Specific psychological triggers that initiate 'appropriate' sinus tachycardia should be considered. As opposed to postural orthostatic tachycardia syndrome (POTS), in which the sinus rate increases with standing upright but does not give rise to supine tachycardia [4], IST is not necessarily, or completely, dependent upon position. An overlap syndrome between IST and POTS is likely [5].

POTS - not tachycardia in supine position.

EPIDEMIOLOGY

The epidemiology of IST remains uncertain since no long-term studies in the modern era have monitored heart rates systematically in the general healthy population to determine which rates are considered 'inappropriate'. What is known about baseline heart rate is that the pulse is regulated via the autonomic nervous system, even at rest, and is gender dependent and age dependent with younger people having higher resting intrinsic (presumed 'chemically denervated') heart rates [6,7]. Commonly, in children, the mean intrinsic rates exceed 120 bpm. The Israeli Cardiovascular Occupational Risk Factors Determination in Israel (CORDIS) study study corroborated that heart rate is inversely related to age, blood pressure elevation and physical activity while heart rate alone is directly, and independently, related to height, coffee drinking and smoking [8].

The prevalence of reported IST may be high with a report suggesting that over 1% of middle-aged individuals meet heart rate criteria [9]. While many may fall under a strict definition of IST based on heart rate alone, without symptoms, this would not necessarily be considered the syndrome of IST. The natural history of the process is not known. Some of the postulated mechanisms are given in **Table 10.2**.

Table 10.2 Possible mechanisms of inappropriate sinus tachycardia	
Considered, but disputed	Autonomic neuropathy Excessive venous pooling α-receptor hyposensitivity Brainstem dysregulation Altered sympathovagal balance
Probable, but poorly understood	Intrinsic sinus node issue β-receptor autoantibodies β-receptor supersensitivity M2 receptor abnormalities Impaired baroreflex control Depressed cardiovagal reflex

MECHANISMS

The causative mechanisms responsible for IST are unclear. There is no reason to suspect just a single cause. In some individuals, the problem is self-limited and short-lived; it can occur after a viral infection and may be related to an inflammatory mediator. For others, it is a long-standing problem.

The sinus node is tightly regulated by the autonomic nervous system and a multiplicity of cardiac channels. Despite the obvious assumption that β-adrenergic stimulation may be a cause for IST, beta-blockers have not proved to be widely effective. Thus, the concept that an intrinsic sinus node process is the cause, even as a developmental process, has taken some hold. Despite evidence of a depressed efferent cardiovagal reflex, and β-adrenergic hypersensitivity, a primary sinus node abnormality has been postulated to be a cause for IST [10].

Two main channels modulate the rate independent of (or interdependent on) the autonomic nervous system: the I_f current and the calcium 'clock'. It remains uncertain which current predominates, but many suspect it is the I_f channel; this mechanism may help understand the value of a specific therapy. In some instances, I_f blockade slows the rate in IST whereas, in others, a calcium channel blocker can be effective.

β-receptor autoantibodies may play a role and be a mechanistic 'breakthrough' [11,12]. Excessive withdrawal of parasympathetic or excitation of the sympathetic nervous system at rest, with exertion, or both, have been implicated. The use of one animal model has suggested a possible role for the right interganglionic nerve and, in another study, the injection of catecholamines into a fat pad containing autonomic ganglia innervating the sino-atrial node was suggested as a possible model for IST [14], but then, any sympathetic stimulation in an animal can cause sinus tachycardia and this is not necessarily inappropriate [15]. No specific animal model can emulate what transpires in humans.

In a report of 24 patients with IST, evaluation included variation in heart rate during slow deep breathing, a 30-to-15 ratio in the heart rate during active standing, the blood pressure response to standing, the cold face test, the Valsalva manoeuvre and the blood pressure response to sustained handgrip each suggested abnormalities in parasympathetic function. Baroreflex gain was reduced. The sympathovagal balance from heart rate variability was preserved, but altered activity in both bands of frequency domain analysis suggested enhanced sinus node automaticity modulated by complex changes in autonomic tone [16]. Other data suggest that IST is related to excess sympathetic activation [4].

Exposure to toxins such as benzene may lead to sinus tachycardia but causative environmental factors remain uncertain. While not the general rule [17], vagal nerve denervation from supraventricular tachycardia ablation can cause IST, at least for a period of time [18–23].

EVALUATION

Before accepting a diagnosis of IST, explicable causes for sinus tachycardia must be meticulously and completely ruled out (**Table 10.1**). There can be confusion regarding the diagnosis and the true cause for tachycardia, such as the case of an undiagnosed infection which may take time to become manifest.

If no cause can be identified, IST is the diagnosis of exclusion, but patients often hang on to this diagnosis as an explanation for symptoms, even if this is not the correct diagnosis and an underlying cause is found. Patients with IST have a multiplicity of symptoms that need to be explored in detail and potentially correlated (or not) with heart rate. Surreptitious drug use and an underlying, undiagnosed condition should be considered. It is necessary to exclude specific physiological and psychological triggers for 'appropriate' sinus tachycardia including exercise, anxiety, panic attacks and pain, to name a few. Anticholinergic drugs, catecholamines, alcohol, caffeine, cocaine, tobacco and beta-blocker withdrawal can increase sinus rate.

It is important to consider and evaluate for POTS. Depending on the patient, besides orthostatic signs as part of the physical examination, an electrocardiogram, and echocardiogram, and potentially a treadmill test or tilt-table test may be required. During the treadmill test, rapid acceleration in heart rate may be seen with minimal exercise, and during a tilt-table test, a gradual increase in heart rate with tilt and little change in blood pressure may indicate POTS. In IST, the heart rate starts off fast but still accelerates rapidly with tilt, perhaps, due to impaired baroreflex gain [24].

Monitoring, at least periodically during symptoms, becomes important to help clinch the diagnosis. It is the most useful approach to correlate palpitations with sinus tachycardia, to determine if sinus tachycardia is the only tachyarrhythmia causing problems and to determine what the rates are and what seems to initiate or trigger this tachycardia. Holter monitoring is considered for patients with daily episodes to correlate symptoms with heart rhythm as well as to document the average heart rate over time. Long-term monitoring to determine the relationship of symptoms to tachycardia or to determine the efficacy of treatment. With advances in implantable loop recorders, this approach may allow for the following of patients and correlation of rate with symptoms as well as providing a guide to treatment.

In most instances, monitoring will provide all required information but for some who have exercise-induced symptoms, a treadmill test can provide additional information. Electrophysiological testing may be useful to determine whether other tachycardias are present, i.e. non-IST tachycardias, which may be playing a role [2].

MANAGEMENT

Managing IST – controlling symptoms and reducing heart rate – remains an ongoing challenge. Heart rate control does not always translate into symptom control. The value of controlling the sinus rate in asymptomatic patients with sinus tachycardia is unknown as any intervention may be worse than the condition itself. In IST, for most patients, no therapy corrects heart rate and symptoms completely and effectively. This is likely to be related to the complexity of the problem and lack of full understanding of causes and mechanisms.

Several case reports, small series and small controlled clinical trials with a short-term follow-up purport to have found treatment solutions. Long-term prospective placebo-controlled clinical trials of any therapeutic intervention are limited. Many treatment recommendations have been made for patients with IST, but these therapies have not been well tested.

Conservative management

A conservative management approach, not utilising any specific therapeutic intervention, but considering lifestyle changes and exercise, as tolerated, is a valuable first step. Exercise may affect more than just the autonomic nervous system – it may affect the I_f channels as well [25]. Effective patient communication and attention seem to improve the outcomes [3].

β-adrenergic blockade

No controlled clinical trial of beta-blockers alone substantiates their use; however, patients with IST may occasionally benefit from beta-blockade [4,26]. Not uncommonly, β-adrenergic blockers, even at high doses, are ineffective and tend to be associated with other symptoms or problems, particularly, if IST is misdiagnosed [27]. Some have suggested that nebivolol may be uniquely effective, but no controlled data support this and a mechanistic explanation is not clear.

Small dosages of benzodiazepines, in addition, may provide relief to patients as it is likely that many patients with IST can have a superimposed anxiety disorder. Fludrocortisone, volume expansion, pressure stockings, phenobarbital, clonidine, psychiatric evaluation, erythropoietin, all recommended by some, have not been proven valuable [5] and these therapies more likely target patients with POTS.

Calcium channel blockade

While the data are weak, a case report has shown benefit in a patient with bronchospastic asthma based on the potential mechanism of sinus tachycardia [28]. Verapamil may be effective and has been recommended but it is generally a second-line drug after a trial of a beta-blocker. Combinations of verapamil and a beta-blocker, while not carefully tested, may be effective.

Ivabradine

Small studies and several case reports (including a patient who developed a cardiomyopathy presumably from IST) have demonstrated the potential value of the I_f blocker, ivabradine, to treat IST [29–37]. Ivabradine can have a dramatic effect on heart rate and can slow it down from a mean of 100 bpm to <75 bpm and the maximum heart rate can slow down from a mean of 160 bpm to 120 bpm. The minimum heart rate can also slow over time.

The efficacy and safety of ivabradine were tested in 18 consecutive symptomatic patients [32]. There was a significant reduction in median and maximal heart rates over 6 months with small changes in minimal heart rate. There was improvement in exercise tolerance.

Phosphene toxicity limited the use of the drug in small numbers of patients, but otherwise, it was well tolerated.

Ivabradine was evaluated in 10 female patients with IST [31]. Ivabradine with a beta-blocker or as sole treatment dramatically and significantly reduced maximum and mean heart rates. Minimum heart rate did not change but symptoms were ameliorated or suppressed in those with a longer-term follow-up [31].

In a report of 20 patients with IST, resistant to beta-blockers or verapamil, titrated doses of metoprolol or ivabradine reduced resting heart rate compared with baseline values. With daily activity, the changes were even more profound, particularly with ivabradine. Ivabradine was well tolerated and most patients were free of symptoms, but metoprolol caused hypotension or bradycardia [26].

In a study of 24 patients with IST, Holter recordings and 36-Item Short Form Health Surveys were performed at 6 months of use. Patients with IST treated with ivabradine showed heart rate normalisation and quality-of-life improvement maintained in the long term. However, discontinuation of this after 1 year unexpectedly showed that the heart rate remained within normal limits in 80% of the patients [38]. The mechanism behind this remains uncertain. It is also not clear which heart rate measure in IST is the most important [26,39].

Ivabradine may also be beneficial after ablation of the slow pathway responsible for atrioventricular (AV) node re-entry after which sinus tachycardia may ensue [30]. In a study of 14 such patients with IST, ivabradine reduced the mean heart rate during daily activity. There was a significant improvement in exercise capacity during treadmill exercise testing on ivabradine [30].

One randomised prospective trial has been completed. In a report of 21 patients with IST randomised to placebo or ivabradine 5 mg twice daily for 6 weeks in a cross-over design, ivabradine eliminated 70% of patients' symptoms (relative risk: 0.25; 95% CI: 0.18–0.34; $P < 0.001$), with 47% of them experiencing complete elimination of symptoms. These effects were associated with a significant reduction of heart rate at rest, with standing and during 24-hour monitoring and during effort. Ivabradine increased exercise performance. No cardiovascular side effects were observed. To date, these are the strongest data we have for any medical intervention for IST [40].

Combinations of metoprolol and ivabradine may be useful. In a report of 20 patients with IST, ivabradine was administered as adjuvant therapy up to 7.5 mg twice daily. While resting, heart rate was similar to metoprolol alone or combination therapy; combined treatment yielded an increase in exercise capacity and a reduction in IST-related symptoms [29].

Ivabradine may precipitate excess bradycardia (especially in combination with beta-blockers or calcium channel blockers) and cause headaches or other minor side effects. Generally, it is well tolerated.

Autonomic denervation

Bilateral stellate ganglion block has been used successfully (with benefit lasting for at least 4 months) in a 34-year old patient with IST unresponsive to medical therapy [41]; the value of complete surgical sympathectomy has not yet been well tested. Innervation may remain via the intrinsic cardiac nervous system. Even complete sympathectomy might not address the primary problem and, therefore, may not successfully treat IST and has potential adverse effects. Further, IST has been observed following heart transplantation even after complete central autonomic denervation [42]. Surgical ablation is not recommended except for the occasional patient who is completely debilitated. The aggressiveness of the surgical therapies that patients are willing to take testifies to the fact that patients with IST can be highly motivated to pursue substantial and risky procedures to eliminate their symptoms.

Sinus node catheter ablation

Radiofrequency ablation to modify the sinus node or eliminate sympathetic inputs is, at best, only partially effective even though early reports suggested ablation had substantial value [3,22,43,44]. Catheter or surgical ablation of the sinus node are now discouraged, even if they are effective, since they do not necessarily improve the outcome of the patients and can cause serious harm, especially if POTS is misdiagnosed as IST (and, as yet, these patients may not even necessarily be that different [4]). For POTS, sinus node ablation will only exacerbate the problem and may lead to hypotension and syncope.

The reports are of small numbers of patients and some testify to good results. In a study of 16 highly symptomatic, drug refractory patients, total sinus node ablation and modification improved heart rates and allowed for chronotropic response in the long term. However, two patients required pacing, one had transient right diaphragmatic paralysis and another had transient superior vena cava syndrome [45].

In another report of 29 patients with IST [44], ablation mapping the earliest site of endocardial activation reduced sinus rates to <90 bpm acutely in 22 patients, progressively in some and abruptly in others. Symptoms recurred a mean of 4.4 months later in 6 of 22 patients but, 3 underwent additional procedures with apparent success.

In a recent report, three-dimensional map-guided ablation of IST was reported in 39 patients [3]. The shift in the earliest sinus node activation site after β-adrenergic blockade was compared with the shift after ablation. Ablation normalised the heart rate but with a more pronounced shift in activation along the crista terminalis than with beta-blockers. Repeat ablation was required in 21% of patients. The authors concluded that adrenergic hypersensitivity is not the only mechanism responsible for IST and that three-dimensional guidance helped to facilitate ablation [3]. In some cases, with a thick terminal crest, an epicardial ablation approach has been utilised [46]. Ablation of the arcuate ridge in a combined epicardial and endocardial approach has been described [43,46].

While we agree that detailed three-dimensional mapping, including, perhaps, the use of noncontact mapping [47], helps to identify sinus nodal sites to ablate in patients with IST, we have observed migrating tachycardia locations with progressive ablation at sites superior to the sinus node in patients with IST. We are not convinced that any three-dimensional mapping approach, even one that utilises unipolar mapping, in an attempt to derive the origin of the sinus node activation, is any better than bipolar mapping.

Such ablation can be fruitless as tachycardia might ultimately come from other sinus nodal sites or from the AV junction after complete sinus node obliteration. This has been observed in surgical ablations and even after sinus node removal. Symptoms can persist despite sinus node slowing and the benefits may be only short term.

Narrowing of the superior vena cava [48], damage to the phrenic nerve [49] and bradycardia requiring need for a pacemaker can occur. Complications may develop days, weeks or months after ablation. Complications are probably being underreported. The possibility of devastating outcomes for an otherwise young healthy person who continues to have symptoms and tachycardia should raise serious concerns about the value of an interventional approach. Patients and referring physicians need to be cognisant that while symptoms may be substantial and patients may be highly motivated, the consequences of aggressive therapeutic attempts may seriously outweigh any potential benefit.

Sinus node surgical ablation

Surgical ablation may be ineffective because in patients with IST, escape rhythms, including those from the AV junction, may also be inappropriately fast. Map-guided total excision of the sinus node has been attempted [50]. Combined epicardial and endocardial ablation approaches have also been attempted with some success [51].

Other methodologies have been utilised to ablate the sinus node surgically, either using a thoracoscopic approach [52], an off-pump beating-heart sinus isolation and ablation through a mini thoracotomy [53] or direct complete removal of the sinus node [50]. Partial cardiac denervation and sinus node ablation have been attempted [54].

CONCLUSION

IST is a poorly defined syndrome which requires the presence of tachycardia, not due to an identifiable underlying cause, plus the presence of symptoms including, but not limited to, weakness, fatigue and palpitations. The potential mechanisms responsible for the syndrome are not well understood. As a result, treatment options are broad, nonspecific and range from various medications to, on rare occasion, when all else fails, radiofrequency ablation.

Key points for clinical practice

A general approach to patients in whom IST is suspected follows:

- Determine if, and when, sinus tachycardia is present, if tachycardia is associated with an explainable cause and/or symptoms and if it is reproducible and persistent under specific conditions. Rule out POTS. Consider psychiatric issues and substance abuse.
- If IST is diagnosed, discuss risks and benefits of any attempted therapy realising that no guideline for treatment is yet established. Symptoms may be independent of heart rate.
- Consider a multidisciplinary-integrated approach to alleviate symptoms and treat heart rate. Effective patient communication and attention seems to improve outcomes [3]. Random and indiscriminate physician referral are of unproven benefit and potentially harmful. The risk of any therapy and its 'nocebo effect' must be weighed against any benefit and the value of any intervention may be dependent upon the relationship to and credibility of the practitioner.
- Encourage graded physical activity as tolerated.
- Eliminate dietary stimulants (e.g. caffeine or alcohol) and stimulant drugs.
- Minimise drug intervention and keep them short term, if possible.
- Treatment begins with modest doses of beta-blockers even though not of proven value. No specific beta-blocker is proven more effective or free of side effects than another.
- Benzodiazepine and beta-blocker combinations, in the hands of an empathetic physician, may be effective. It is likely that many patients with IST have a superimposed anxiety disorder.
- Ivabradine 5.0–7.5 mg twice daily may work, yet it is not approved in the United States. Combinations with metoprolol appear effective if ivabradine alone is not.
- Radiofrequency ablation should be considered only if sinus rates are extremely fast, the patient has IST with symptoms due to tachycardia, and all other therapies failed. This is the option of last resort and not encouraged.

REFERENCES

1. Rubenstein JC, Freher M, Kadish A, Goldberger JJ. Diurnal heart rate patterns in inappropriate sinus tachycardia. Pacing Clin Electrophysiol 2010; 33:911–919.
2. Frankel DS, Lin D, Anastasio N, et al. Frequent additional tachyarrhythmias in patients with inappropriate sinus tachycardia undergoing sinus node modification: an important cause of symptom recurrence. J Cardiovasc Electrophysiol 2012; 23:835–839.
3. Marrouche NF, Beheiry S, Tomassoni G, et al. Three-dimensional nonfluoroscopic mapping and ablation of inappropriate sinus tachycardia. Procedural strategies and long-term outcome. J Am Coll Cardiol 2002; 39:1046–1054.
4. Nwazue VC, Paranjape SY, Black BK, et al. Postural tachycardia syndrome and inappropriate sinus tachycardia: role of autonomic modulation and sinus node automaticity. J Am Heart Assoc 2014; 3:e000700.
5. Brady PA, Low PA, Shen WK. Inappropriate sinus tachycardia, postural orthostatic tachycardia syndrome, and overlapping syndromes. Pacing Clin Electrophysiol 2005; 28:1112–1121.
6. Jose AD, Collison D. The normal range and determinants of the intrinsic heart rate in man. Cardiovasc Res 1970; 4:160–167.
7. Marcus B, Gillette PC, Garson A Jr. Intrinsic heart rate in children and young adults: an index of sinus node function isolated from autonomic control. Am Heart J 1990; 119:911–916.
8. Kristal-Boneh E, Harari G, Weinstein Y, Green MS. Factors affecting differences in supine, sitting, and standing heart rate: the Israeli CORDIS study. Aviat Space Environ Med 1995; 66:775–779.
9. Still AM, Raatikainen P, Ylitalo A, et al. Prevalence, characteristics and natural course of inappropriate sinus tachycardia. Europace 2005; 7:104–112.
10. Morillo CA, Klein GJ, Thakur RK, et al. Mechanism of 'inappropriate' sinus tachycardia. Role of sympathovagal balance. Circulation 1994; 90:873–877.
11. Chiale PA, Garro HA, Schmidberg J, et al. Inappropriate sinus tachycardia may be related to an immunologic disorder involving cardiac beta andrenergic receptors. Heart Rhythm 2006; 3:1182–1186.
12. Nattel S. Inappropriate sinus tachycardia and beta-receptor autoantibodies: A mechanistic breakthrough? Heart Rhythm 2006; 3:1187–1188.
13. Zhou J, Scherlag BJ, Niu G, et al. Anatomy and physiology of the right interganglionic nerve: Implications for the pathophysiology of inappropriate sinus tachycardia. J Cardiovasc Electrophysiol 2008; 19:971–976.
14. Scherlag BJ, Yamanashi WS, Amin R, Lazzara R, Jackman WM. Experimental model of inappropriate sinus tachycardia: Initiation and ablation. J Interv Card Electrophysiol 2005; 13:21–29.
15. Olshansky B. What's so inappropriate about sinus tachycardia? J Cardiovasc Electrophysiol 2008; 19:977–978.
16. Ptaszynski P, Kaczmarek K, Klingenheben T, et al. Noninvasive assessment of autonomic cardiovascular activity in patients with inappropriate sinus tachycardia. Am J Cardiol 2013; 112:811–815.
17. Purerfellner H, Mascherbauer R, Nesser HJ. Absence of significant changes in heart rate variability after slow pathway ablation of AV nodal reentrant tachycardia by using serial holter recordings. Am Heart J 1998; 136:259–263.
18. Ehlert FA, Goldberger JJ, Brooks R, Miller S, Kadish AH. Persistent inappropriate sinus tachycardia after radiofrequency current catheter modification of the atrioventricular node. Am J Cardiol 1992; 69:1092–1095.
19. Kocovic DZ, Harada T, Shea JB, Soroff D, Friedman PL. Alterations of heart rate and of heart rate variability after radiofrequency catheter ablation of supraventricular tachycardia. Delineation of parasympathetic pathways in the human heart. Circulation 1993; 88:1671–1681.
20. Skeberis V, Simonis F, Tsakonas K, et al. Inappropriate sinus tachycardia following radiofrequency ablation of AV nodal tachycardia: Incidence and clinical significance. Pacing Clin Electrophysiol 1994; 17:924–927.
21. Adler A, Rosso R, Meir I, Viskin S. Ivabradine for the prevention of inappropriate shocks due to sinus tachycardia in patients with an implanted cardioverter defibrillator. Europace 2013; 15:362–365.
22. Skeberis V, Simonis F, Tsakonas K, et al. Inappropriate sinus tachycardia following radiofrequency ablation of AV nodal tachycardia: Incidence and clinical significance. Pacing Clin Electrophysiol 1994; 17:924–927.
23. Moreira JM, Curimbaba J, Filho HC, Pimenta J. Persistent inappropriate sinus tachycardia after radiofrequency ablation of left lateral accessory pathway. J Cardiovasc Electrophysiol 2006; 17:678–681.
24. Leon H, Guzman JC, Kuusela T, et al. Impaired baroreflex gain in patients with inappropriate sinus tachycardia. J Cardiovasc Electrophysiol 2005; 16:64–68.

25. D'Souza A, Bucchi A, Johnsen AB, et al. Exercise training reduces resting heart rate via downregulation of the funny channel HCN4. Nat Commun 2014; 5:3775.

26. Ptaszynski P, Kaczmarek K, Ruta J, Klingenheben T, Wranicz JK. Metoprolol succinate vs. ivabradine in the treatment of inappropriate sinus tachycardia in patients unresponsive to previous pharmacological therapy. Europace 2013; 15:116–121.

27. De Pauw M, Tromp F, De Buyzere M. Sinus tachycardia: don't blame the whistle-blower. Acta Cardiol 2013; 68:315–317.

28. Foster MC, Levine PA. Use of verapamil to control an inappropriate chronic sinus tachycardia. Chest 1984; 85:697–699.

29. Ptaszynski P, Kaczmarek K, Ruta J, et al. Ivabradine in combination with metoprolol succinate in the treatment of inappropriate sinus tachycardia. J Cardiovasc Pharmacol Ther 2013; 18:338–344.

30. Ptaszynski P, Kaczmarek K, Ruta J, Klingenheben T, Wranicz JK. Ivabradine in the treatment of inappropriate sinus tachycardia in patients after successful radiofrequency catheter ablation of atrioventricular node slow pathway. Pacing Clin Electrophysiol 2013; 36:42–49.

31. Zellerhoff S, Hinterseer M, Felix Krull B, et al. Ivabradine in patients with inappropriate sinus tachycardia. Naunyn Schmiedebergs Arch Pharmacol 2010; 382:483–486.

32. Calo L, Rebecchi M, Sette A, et al. Efficacy of ivabradine administration in patients affected by inappropriate sinus tachycardia. Heart Rhythm 2010; 7:1318–1323.

33. Kaplinsky E, Comes FP, Urondo LS, Ayma FP. Efficacy of ivabradine in four patients with inappropriate sinus tachycardia: a three month-long experience based on electrocardiographic, holter monitoring, exercise tolerance and quality of life assessments. Cardiol J 2010; 17:166–171.

34. Schulze V, Steiner S, Hennersdorf M, Strauer BE. Ivabradine as an alternative therapeutic trial in the therapy of inappropriate sinus tachycardia: a case report. Cardiology 2008; 110:206–208.

35. Kumar Goyal V, Godara S, Chandra Sadasukhi T, Lal Gupta H. Management of inappropriate sinus tachycardia with ivabradine in a renal transplant recipient. Drug Discov Ther 2014; 8:132–133.

36. Winum PF, Cayla G, Rubini M, Beck L, Messner-Pellenc P. A case of cardiomyopathy induced by inappropriate sinus tachycardia and cured by ivabradine. Pacing Clin Electrophysiol 2009; 32:942–944.

37. Weyn T, Stockman D, Degreef Y. The use of ivabradine for inappropriate sinus tachycardia. Acta Cardiol 2011; 66:259–262.

38. Benezet-Mazuecos J, Rubio JM, Farre J, et al. Long-term outcomes of ivabradine in inappropriate sinus tachycardia patients: Appropriate efficacy or inappropriate patients. Pacing Clin Electrophysiol 2013; 36:830–836.

39. Wichterle D. Ivabradine for inappropriate sinus tachycardia: Another piece of evidence. Europace 2013; 15:9–10.

40. Cappato R, Castelvecchio S, Ricci C, et al. Clinical efficacy of ivabradine in patients with inappropriate sinus tachycardia: a prospective, randomized, placebo-controlled, double-blind, crossover evaluation. J Am Coll Cardiol 2012; 60:1323–1329.

41. Huang HD, Tamarisa R, Mathur N, et al. Stellate ganglion block: a therapeutic alternative for patients with medically refractory inappropriate sinus tachycardia? J Electrocardiol 2013; 46:693–696.

42. Ho RT, Ortman M, Mather PJ, Rubin S. Inappropriate sinus tachycardia in a transplanted heart – further insights into pathogenesis. Heart Rhythm 2011; 8:781–783.

43. Killu AM, Syed FF, Wu P, Asirvatham SJ. Refractory inappropriate sinus tachycardia successfully treated with radiofrequency ablation at the arcuate ridge. Heart Rhythm 2012; 9:1324–1327.

44. Man KC, Knight B, Tse HF, et al. Radiofrequency catheter ablation of inappropriate sinus tachycardia guided by activation mapping. J Am Coll Cardiol 2000; 35:451–457.

45. Lee RJ, Kalman JM, Fitzpatrick AP, et al. Radiofrequency catheter modification of the sinus node for 'inappropriate' sinus tachycardia. Circulation 1995; 92:2919–2928.

46. Koplan BA, Parkash R, Couper G, Stevenson WG. Combined epicardial–endocardial approach to ablation of inappropriate sinus tachycardia. J Cardiovasc Electrophysiol 2004; 15:237–240.

47. Takemoto M, Mukai Y, Inoue S, et al. Usefulness of non-contact mapping for radiofrequency catheter ablation of inappropriate sinus tachycardia: new procedural strategy and long-term clinical outcome. Intern Med 2012; 51:357–362.

48. Callans DJ, Ren JF, Schwartzman D, et al. Narrowing of the superior vena cava-right atrium junction during radiofrequency catheter ablation for inappropriate sinus tachycardia: analysis with intracardiac echocardiography. J Am Coll Cardiol 1999; 33:1667–1670.

49. Vatasescu R, Shalganov T, Kardos A, et al. Right diaphragmatic paralysis following endocardial cryothermal ablation of inappropriate sinus tachycardia. Europace 2006; 8:904–906.

50. Selten K, Van Brakel TJ, Van Swieten HA, Smeets JL. Mapping-guided total excision of the sinoatrial node for inappropriate sinus tachycardia. J Thorac Cardiovasc Surg 2014; 147:e56–e58.
51. Jacobson JT, Kraus A, Lee R, Goldberger JJ. Epicardial/endocardial sinus node ablation after failed endocardial ablation for the treatment of inappropriate sinus tachycardia. J Cardiovasc Electrophysiol 2014; 25:236–241.
52. Beaver TM, Miles WM, Conti JB, et al. Minimally invasive ablation of a migrating focus of inappropriate sinus tachycardia. J Thorac Cardiovasc Surg 2010; 139:506–507.
53. Kreisel D, Bailey M, Lindsay BD, Damiano RJ Jr. A minimally invasive surgical treatment for inappropriate sinus tachycardia. J Thorac Cardiovasc Surg 2005; 130:598–599.
54. Taketani T, Wolf RK, Garrett JV. Partial cardiac denervation and sinus node modification for inappropriate sinus tachycardia. Ann Thorac Surg 2007; 84:652–654.

Index

Note: Page numbers in **bold** or *italic* refer to tables or figures, respectively.